Nourish the Flame Within

A Guide to Connecting to the Human Soul for Reiki, Martial Arts and Life.

By Lynette Avis and David Brown

AuthorHouse™
1663 Liberty Drive
Bloomington, IN 47403
www.authorhouse.com
Phone: 1-800-839-8640

Published by AuthorHouse 04/11/2013

ISBN: 978-1-4772-5083-9 (sc)
978-1-4772-5098-3 (e)

Any people depicted in stock imagery provided by Thinkstock are models,
and such images are being used for illustrative purposes only.
Certain stock imagery © Thinkstock.

This book is printed on acid-free paper.

authorHOUSE®

Acknowledgements

We would like to say a huge thank you to all of the people who have helped in the writing of this book. They have given their time, insights, and opinions which have been very helpful to us. We would like to give a special thank you to Janette Marshall for sharing her work and knowledge with us and for allowing us to reproduce her vibration exercise in this book. We would also like to say thank you to those people who allowed us to use photographs of them in this book.

Thank you all.

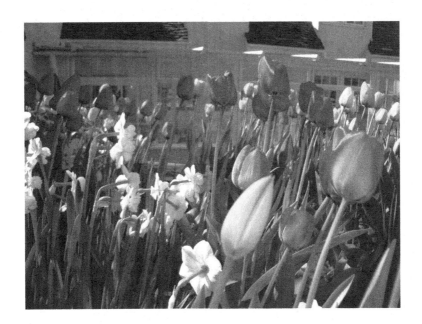

This book is dedicated to Rachael

We have stopped for a moment to encounter each other, to meet, to love, to share.
This is a precious moment, but it is transient. It is a little parenthesis in eternity.
If we share with caring, light-heartedness, and love, we will create abundance
and joy for each other. And then this moment will have been worthwhile.

—Deepak Chopra

We the authors of this book wish it to be known that all of the ideas and beliefs discussed within this book are our own personal opinions. They are not the opinions or beliefs of any other person or organisation to which we may be connected.

We have included the exercises and meditations within this book with the purpose of allowing all who wish to do so the opportunity to experience many forms of energetic engagement and encounter. There is a great deal to be gained from doing any of the exercises and meditations. It is the individual's personal choice, responsibility and decision as to which meditations and exercises they wish to use from this book. All of the meditations and exercises are included for specific purposes. For example the health meditations will help to improve your health and vitality and the self-growth and life awareness meditations will help develop your relationship with self and others.

The first meditation "Direct communication with spirit energy" is designed to do what it says. It will bring the person in direct contact with spirit energy. As the book will go onto explain there are many different forms of energy and spirit energy is just one of those forms. Living people are spirit energy and that spirit energy remains in existence when the physical body dies and decays.

Doing this particular meditation will develop the individual's ability to communicate with spirit energy and this contact may take many forms. It may be that the individual will experience seeing spirit, hearing spirit and feeling spirit. No one can predict how the path to spirit communication will open for any individual. Therefore we recommend that to walk this path the individual may wish to do so with the help of a qualified medium who is knowledgeable about the subject of spiritual communication. The individual engaging in the exercises or meditations must take full responsibility for all outcomes resulting from doing any exercise or meditation given within this book.

Contents

A Warm Welcome from Lynette........

I am so pleased that you have found this book. It has been written with sharing in mind. What you will find within the pages of this book may well be a new way of looking at life and the universe for you. We have both written all that is within this book with both love and care. We hope that you find something of use to you.

We have tried to give two perspectives—both the scientific and the mystic view of energy. What you may well find is that they are not so different. David takes you on a journey through science to discuss and discover some of the latest and most recent thinking on what has made the universe. I take you to all sorts of places within your mind, your energy, your thoughts, your feelings, and your memories. I teach you to connect to the place beyond this life through the use of meditation and to connect to yourself and others. We discuss your health and well-being, your spiritual body, and your life and your connection to life.

This book is a tool for life; it has been written with the intention of sharing our knowledge with you. I would like to think that no matter who reads this book, he or she will find something of use. This book is a book of wisdom and balance, and we have drawn that wisdom from many sources. We have drawn on the wisdom of wise men and women, on nature, and on the Universe itself to bring this book to you.

We are not all the same, although we are all human beings. We are individuals, and we all have varying though similar needs within life itself. Both David and I as individuals are similar in many of our beliefs and understandings, but we are two individuals, and we have tried to bring to you a balanced perspective by looking at this subject through two people's eyes—two people's eyes who view life differently, one a trained artist and designer and the other a trained scientist. David and I use the opposite sides of our brains to view life. By doing so, we hope to have catered for most people. Well, I leave you now to start on this journey with us. I am so excited for you.

Please enjoy the experience.

Lynette

XXX

This book deals with life and the fundamental issues that make your life work. It looks at you and your life through the perspective of Universal Energy. It touches on issues that have a relationship to you and your life. Very often we find ourselves at odds with other people and life itself. This leaves us feeling vulnerable and alone. Within the pages of this book we help you, through the use of meditation, Universal Energy, and wisdom, to look at yourself and your life.

We do this in a way that you may find to be a new perspective and a new way of looking at Reality in general and your own reality in particular. We give you the tools to deal with your daily life and your health and well-being, and we help you to make changes within your life for the better. We start this journey through science by understanding how the Universe connects to you and you to it through energy. Within this book, we learn how by the use of meditations we can connect to the Universe and harness the Universal Energy that is freely available to all, including you. We touch on how to meditate, what meditation is, and how we can use it in many ways for many things in the pursuit of a better us. This takes us to martial arts and Reiki—how we can connect to the Universal Energy for the enhancement of those practices and how they can help you in your life.

To understand the essence of this book, we have to grasp a different way of looking at the world. It is Reality; it is not the way we are used to experiencing reality or even thinking about reality. Great minds in the twentieth century discovered that energy is the essence of the universe. For hundreds of years, scientists have tried to break matter and reality down into smaller and smaller particles in the hope of finding the particle or particles that are the essence of it all. What they found was emptiness, a void filled with vibrancy, a description more in keeping with the mystic teachings of the East than the conclusions of Western science. Quantum physics seemed to be describing a reality that had been taught by the cultures of Hinduism, Buddhism, Zen, Taoism, and the like for centuries, even millennia. It pointed to a reality that is beyond the particle model that we once believed was the truth, a description that built reality up from an intangible emptiness without matter and form, into a reality that is still dynamic and powerful and yet unarguably solid and with shape and structure.

It is easy to see how Western science made the error, as our senses point to a separation between things. We sense that objects have discrete boundaries and that things start and finish. Your eyes tell you that you are separate from the chair you are sitting in and the book you are reading. Modern science now tells us that if we break matter down enough, we have simply energy. Both quantum physics and the East describe this energy as a quantum soup from which all things come. It is like a void that is not empty but, rather, is full of nothingness, or—to use a phrase that is in keeping with this book—*energy with undefined potential*. This is how it all began, and in the science chapter of this book we will discuss how this process might have come about. In its many forms, this undefined energy has evolved and changed, building on generation after generation, becoming more and more defined, and yet inextricably connected to the undefined whole. This process has taken place as conditions have allowed, for every configuration can only exist as the energy allows it to exist. The apparent harshness of nature is that things are formed and then they perish, existing only while conditions make it possible. For us as humans, life is this most treasured and tenuous thread, along which the energy of life flows. Once the energy stops flowing, that defined potential ceases to exist and becomes part of the whole, the void, the energy with undefined potential.

Our minds are able to harness this energy consciously as it flows along the thread, which has led to the creation of poets, artists, scientists, and visionaries who have contributed to the wealth of beauty and understanding in art, the written word, science and technology, philosophy and ethics, religion, and culture. Through our thoughts, we have harnessed the power of the mind and made our dreams reality -as well as our nightmares. Some people intuitively seem to know how this process works and are incredibly productive, creative, and effective in their lives. Some of these people, such as Dickens, Austen, Shakespeare, and Shaw, wrote great works of literature, while others, such as Mozart, Beethoven, Monet, and Van Gogh, create masterpieces in art and music. Richard Branson, John D. Rockefeller and Alan Sugar have a natural flare and success in business, while Gandhi, Martin Luther King, Steve Jobs, and Abraham Lincoln had skills in leadership and motivation. Still others, including Morihei Ueshiba, Yamaoka Tesshu, and Bruce Lee, have been motivated to follow paths that unleashed their potential through martial arts, while others seek that potential through healing, such as Mother Teresa, Mikao Usui, and Betty Shine.

There are countless examples of people throughout history who have felt their own inner power lead them to follow a path that made them feel fulfilled and empowered, but this need not be the state of the privileged few but something that we can all enjoy and feel privileged to take part in. We need to learn how to harness this conscious control of Energy and use it for the betterment of ourselves and others, so that we may contribute something worthwhile to those around us and to society at large. We help our readers do this by giving them the tools by which they can achieve change to themselves and their life. We give personal encouragement to the reader and positive ways of looking at any situation for positive outcomes to that situation.

Within this book are contained fourteen methods of meditation that allow us to consciously harness energy through meditation, methods that will help to empower us and help us live a more fulfilling and meaningful existence. These are tools for life, tools that can be used throughout our lives.

The first three of these meditations in chapter 2 of this book bring us into connection with the quantum soup, that which has been present since the beginning and has created the universe, the stars, the planets, and life itself. It feels expansive, energising, calming, and revitalizing.

To complement the first set of meditations, we have included three meditations relating to health. These three meditations can be found in chapter 3, the "health" chapter of this book. They will help to dispel negative energy and help to concentrate positive energy in the body, keeping that energy healthy and flowing. They are the second set of meditations.

We also have three meditations to connect us to the energy that is "you"—that part of the Universe that is you—creating a sense of what you truly are. They are the third set of meditations and can be found in chapter 4.

We have a final group of meditations that show you how the energy that is "you" can be used in the world, helping to make the "you" energy more interactive with the whole. Through your thoughts, actions, ideas, and emotions, "you" interact with the world around you, influencing and affecting it as it, in turn, influences and affects you. These meditations can be found in the fifth chapter of the book.

These twelve meditations come to us from extensive work in these areas and have been of great value to us. The last two meditations are martial arts and Reiki healing. Over many years we have extensive experience in these forms of meditation, in which the stillness of meditation has brought us to the realization of the Energy that creates us, surrounds us, and is within us. Passionate about these subjects, we have become lovers of life itself, a sense that we are truly alive and part of something magnificent. To do this and keep doing it requires commitment and dedication, a passion to invest in this wonderful gift we call life. We simply wish to share this with others, and we do so in our daily lives. This book is an extension of that desire. If we can harness this energy within us and all around us, we can consciously make the lives we want for ourselves. It can be abused, as all things can be abused, but we hope that it will be used for good to help all that read it, and that they *in turn* will help others.

What is unique about this book is that it touches on subjects that are usually considered mystical, simply experiential, and without any scientific backing or rigor. What we have tried to do is incorporate the accumulated knowledge of science, mysticism, self-development, and self-study to show that there is a meeting point that both worlds share that can help to improve our understanding and experience of both, that the experiences people have in meditation and through years of self-study actually have a basis in scientific theory, and that the observations in science are connected to our daily living experience. In short, what is often considered mystical is in fact very natural and can be explained through science. Having said that, our understanding in science is limited, and there are holes in our knowledge that will be filled in time. Similarly, there are holes in our experience as individuals and as a species. The subject of this book is a work in progress, and science cannot explain all there is to explain. Einstein tried to unify all things in a scientifically and mathematically sound way and was unable to do so in his lifetime. We must be patient, and in time we will discover the answers. In the meantime, this is an attempt to draw these two worlds together, based upon our understanding, knowledge and experience.

What makes us qualified to take on such a book? Both Lynette and I have a passion for life and people, a desire to share that which we have experienced through our lives with others in the hope that it has some benefit and use to them. Life is about sharing experience and knowledge, as that is how the human species evolves.

Education is an admirable thing, but it is well to remember from time to time that nothing that is worth knowing can be taught.

—Oscar Wilde

What we wish to do is open people up to the possibility that they can touch and be part of something greater, to allow people to experience that which cannot be taught. How many of us give a moment's thought as to the nature of truth, energy or reality? How should we think about it and in what context? We are included in the Universe and we are also included in Energy and Reality. Just as universe is often thought of as out there or out of reach and energy is thought of as separate from us, so reality is a personal perspective on a larger Truth.

We have discovered so much within our journeys in martial arts, Reiki, and meditation through experiencing their wonder and magnificence. So let us share: let us take you on a journey through science and experience that points to Reality. There is much to be discovered and that will be done by you. Maybe you will develop a love of meditation or Reiki or even martial arts, but really it is about discovering a love of yourself and your life and your place in it. We wish you well on your journey, and so let us now discover together…

All life is an experiment. The more experiments you make the better.

—Ralph Waldo Emerson

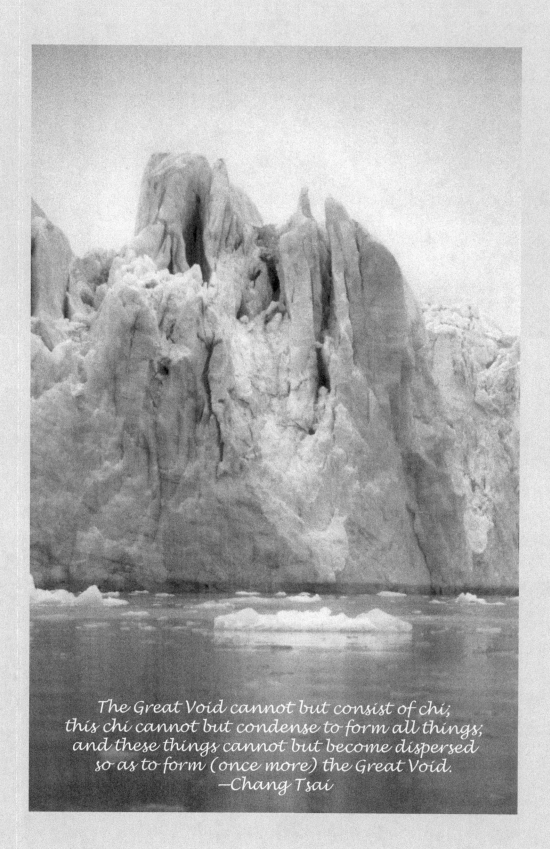

The Great Void cannot but consist of chi;
this chi cannot but condense to form all things;
and these things cannot but become dispersed
so as to form (once more) the Great Void.
                    —Chang Tsai

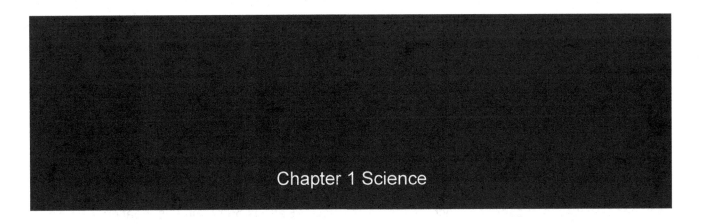

Energy Science

One of the many defining moments in the journey of scientific discovery was Einstein's realisation and rationalisation of his famous equation $E = mc^2$, and many of the ideas that have sprung from this insight. In essence, this equation describes Reality. It explains that Energy is the essence of all things. It points to the reality that matter and the means by which matter interacts are all manifestations of energy.

The idea of the quantum field and superstring theory has taken this concept a stage further. By this theory, scientists recognise that this Energy is everywhere, a continuous medium throughout the cosmos that condenses to create form or matter and disperses to create the "emptiness" of space. This is a dynamic system, in which matter spontaneously forms and disappears and Energy flows along paths of Nature's creation. As Energy flows, it creates electrons, protons, and neutrons, the atoms of the elements and the molecules that are created by the interaction of these elements. These in turn go on to create galaxies, suns, planets, and moons. This Energy flows to create life and to generate the wind and the clouds, as well as thunder and lightning of summer storms. It creates man, and it is the essence of the thoughts and innovations of the human race. It is the force behind nature, it is the force of nature, and it is this flowing quality that has led us to where we are today. Without flow, nature does not move on—it cannot evolve and it will not change. As one thing changes, so the things with which it interacts change, generating a pulsing, thriving, living Universe that is constantly in a state of flux.

The Way Energy Flows

Nothing is in isolation. Scientifically, man has tried to explain this through the laws of thermodynamics, which is the study of the flow of heat (energy). There are four laws, which we will describe in relation to energy, rather than to heat alone, so that it is relevant to the book.

Law 0 states that heat will not flow between objects of the same temperature. In short, the universe seeks to keep itself in balance. Heat moves from a warmer towards a colder object, just as air moves from a high pressure to a low pressure, creating winds and weather systems. So it is with all energy. It flows where nature directs it, where nature has need of it. If all is in balance, energy has no need to flow anywhere. It holds its position in space. All is calm like a very hot summer's day. The air is motionless. Every leaf on every tree is still, no bird sings, and all you really want to do is lie still, quiet, sipping a beer or a cocktail. On a blustery or stormy day, the wind rages to seek balance, and children charge around the park, kicking up the autumn leaves as if affected by the imbalance around them. After the storm, all is still and calm. Nature swings in and out of balance like a pendulum, rarely finding true equilibrium, but rather moving constantly towards it and away from it in an endless cycle of interacting systems seeking balance. In man's desire to be comfortable and cosseted, he removes the impulse for imbalance and therefore the drive for growth. He shrinks away from uncertainty and the unpredictability of life itself. This is indeed the wave upon which mankind can surf, driving him to create art, science, technology, innovations, and levels of understanding once undreamed of. It is this that has driven the universe to evolve beyond its original heat and gas. Imbalance has been the driving force behind it all, because energy needs to have a reason to flow. Achieving balance is the reason, but more on that and chaos theory later.

Law 1 states heat (energy) cannot be created or destroyed. (This is also known as the law of conservation of energy.) Heat can only flow from place to place or change form. You have a pot of water at room temperature. You add some heat to the system. First, the temperature and energy of the water increases. Second, the system releases some energy and it works on the environment (maybe heating the air around the water, making the air rise). The same principle operates throughout the universe. The sun generates electromagnetic energy through the fusion reactions that take place due to its immense heat, sending waves of energy out across the solar system. Earth is bathed in this, heating the air and the ground. Plants use the energy to photosynthesise, and animals on the planet eat the plants and each other to convert that food energy into heat and power for movement. This never-ending cycle of recycling energy is the reason there is life on earth.

Law 2 discusses entropy, or disorder. With added heat there is an increase in disorder. At the Big Bang the universe was highly disordered. As the temperature fell, a greater and greater order was established across the universe. Even today there are pockets of disorder in the universe in the form of the many stars that are immensely hot, so hot in fact that they can split and fuse the atoms within them, making new elements and destroying old ones. This is a highly volatile and unstable system, in constant flux, undergoing endless change. Even the earth has disorder, enough for change, but things are more stable here, enough for life. Again, this is another order of balance, another way in which energy can flow.

Law 3 states that 100% efficiency is impossible. Since 100% efficiency is impossible, it means that there are no truly reversible processes. That in turn means that all processes are irreversible. For every interaction, the universe is changed forever. This assures the evolution of the universe. Energy leaks out of systems into other systems, making all systems interrelated and interconnected. The vast network of interconnectedness means that we cannot truly know all the consequences of our actions and how these actions can seep into other streams of consciousness. We cannot truly know the good we can do. We also cannot truly know the harm we can do. We must strive to be at peace and walk with peaceful steps through our lives. The energy of our thoughts and actions may have far reaching consequences. The least we can do is be kind. By connecting to the force of this energy, maybe we are led to our destiny.

Unravelling the Energy of the Universe

As scientists discover concepts to describe their observations, we must realise that these concepts cannot fully describe this living universe of energy. It describes things as best we can for the moment, until we have the next piece of the jigsaw that clarifies understanding and brings reality into sharper focus. For thousands of years scientists and philosophers have sought out the indivisible particles that make up the universe. The discovery of the atom was hailed as a landmark on this journey, until evidence pointed to the fact that atoms themselves were made up of smaller particles. Nature unfurled her secrets piecemeal. First the electron and then the proton and neutron were revealed, leading to experimental evidence that was in conflict with the foundations of classical physics. Thus quantum physics was born, an explanation of reality at the subatomic level, where things are so small and move so fast that Newton's classical explanations of reality just do not work. A new view began to be revealed that pointed away from the solid nature of particles and into the more fluid and dynamic realm of waves. The idea of particles seemed indeed to be an illusion, a concept adopted by man due to his limited understanding and conceptualisation of the truth.

Deeper and deeper man probed into reality, until he reached the understanding that electrons were best described as clouds, with no perceptible outer edge *per se*, but rather the probability of being in a certain place at a particular time. By association, this means that atoms do not really have a discrete outer edge either, simply a sphere of influence that allows interactions with other atoms as conditions permit. Electromagnetic force holds electrons around the nucleus of an atom. Electrons are negatively charged, while the protons in the nucleus of an atom are positively charged, generating an electromagnetic attraction. Electrons, held relatively close to the nucleus, are confined in a small space, and because of the nature of energy, they must move. They move so fast, in fact, that they create the illusion that an atom has a solid edge.

It is theorised that protons and neutrons themselves are made up of quarks. A single quark has yet to be isolated, but evidence points to quarks interacting in threes, the combination of quarks determining whether a proton or a neutron is created. Protons and neutrons are confined within the nucleus by the strong nuclear force. Energy must move, so the protons and neutrons spin in their confinement, creating the illusion of a discrete nucleus. Quarks are also held tight by the strong nuclear force, causing them to spin as well. The smaller the confinement, the greater the speed, and it is the nature of these interactions, such as electromagnetism and the strong nuclear force, that forces these confinements and so allows such speeds to be reached. This creates the illusion of solidity and particles. Think of a fast flowing waterfall. To the eye, it appears as a whole and solid column, when in reality there are gaps between the water droplets and water molecules. Touch the falling water, and you will feel it very much as a solid object as the force of the water in motion interacts with you.

The energies of these protons, neutrons, electrons, and atoms are so great, just like the fast flowing waterfall, that they seem impossible to penetrate. On earth, temperatures and speeds are such that these particles are more or less immutable. The science of chemistry is the study of the interaction between elements and the complex bonds that are formed between the electrons of interacting atoms. It goes to explain much of our physical world, while the realm of biology seeks to explain the interaction of these molecules in living systems. What we must never forget is that these molecules are made up of atoms that are themselves made up of these fast-spinning quarks, protons, neutrons, and electrons.

It is physics in all its wondrous branches that studies the nature of reality at the nuclear level. Given enough energy, the nucleus can be penetrated and its phenomenal energy unleashed. It is this energy that creates the heat from the sun. Millions of nuclei collide each second, fusing together to create new elements. This cannot be achieved without the immense heat that comes from having so many nuclei so tightly packed together under such pressure from gravity. On earth we have harnessed the power of nuclear fusion to create power stations and bombs, and for many years we have tried to use nuclear fission to generate a clean power source.

We have also managed to gain access to the energy within these fundamental particles by accelerating them to near light speeds and smashing them together. Laboratories such as Fermilab or the Large Hadron Collider at CERN demonstrate that these particles do not have other particles inside them, but rather they come together to create new ones, a product of the energy within them and the energy of the speed at which they travel. All manner of particles have been discovered, but rather than being smaller constituents of a larger particle, they are in fact a spontaneous manifestation of the energy within the process. In short, it is energy taking physical form, a clue perhaps to the process involved in the forming of the universe after the Big Bang.

In the beginning, all was dark. All of the universe was confined into an infinitely small space of infinite weight and infinite gravity, until it began to expand outward in a process we now refer to as the Big Bang. The universe was phenomenal heat expanding at rapid speed, surging tides of energy as yet too hot to have form. As it cooled, the universe began to take shape, energy taking form as quarks and leptons at first, then coalescing into protons and neutrons, and later still into atoms. These atoms were simply hydrogen and helium, scattered across the universe in such volumes that the effect of gravity began slowly to work its magic. Massive clouds began to form that packed tighter and tighter until stars ignited in the universe, the melting pots that would become the birthplace of the ninety-two naturally occurring elements that would ultimately make life possible on earth.

Beauty, Evolution, and Change

As the universe has evolved, so the uses to which energy has been put have diversified. The high-energy furnaces of the stars are still being born and are dying today, continuing the process of recycling generation after generation. But with every generation, something new is created—a small step forward that guarantees that the universe will never be the same again. The nature of energy is to flow, as if it is seeking the way forward, and with every new thing that is created, energy has something new to work with to create the next new thing. Energy interacting with itself created the physical universe, with this vitality woven into the very fabric of reality. This vitality assures change, which means the universe is certain to evolve and move on. Energy's vitality ensures a chaotic aspect to the universe, but that does not mean there is no order.

Man has intuitively recognised the beauty that is inherent in nature. Leonardo da Vinci investigated our sense of beauty and harmony and called it the "golden section". He used it in many of his paintings, as did Michelangelo and other great artists, architects, sculptors, and perhaps even musicians. Even before da Vinci's research, ancient Egyptians appear to have used the golden section to build the pyramids, while the ancient Greeks used it to create the proportions of the Parthenon. What is fascinating is that the proportions of the golden section, a ratio of 1:1.618, appear in nature over and over again, not just in living things like the structure of the nautilus shell, the shape of the perfectly proportioned human face, DNA, and the branching patterns in trees, but also in inanimate structures such as galaxies, river tributaries, the solar system, and even the curves of waves.

Built into that order is the chance for change, adaptation, and evolution. The sperm and egg that came together to create you were alive, each with a unique genetic combination achieved by the recombination of DNA during the process of making them, leading to a still more unique genetic combination when they joined to create you. Time and again, nature creates opportunities for uniqueness; each one of us is an example of that. But even before life appeared in the universe, that same principle—that same uniqueness that creates something unique—ensures that the universe can never be the same again. It creates without purpose. It creates because that is what it does. In man's desire to learn and understand, he has tried to predict the chaotic nature of energy and has devised chaos theory, which demonstrates the order and pattern behind the seemingly random behaviour of nature. Darwin described a similar principle in *On the Origin of Species* and called it evolution. Only natural selection ensures the survival of individuals, but it is the built-in, seemingly random change of nature that creates the myriad beauty and wonder in the universe we are able to witness today.

It is as if energy is a pioneer, always looking for a new path to reveal new levels of potential. And look at what energy has achieved in the universe up until now. That is not to say that energy thinks or has conscious thought, but rather it acts according to its nature, and its nature is flow, vitality, power, and potential. It finds the path of possibility and makes it real. In man, energy does think and does have conscious thought. Man has this incredible capability to guide and influence energy through thought as well as action.

Man's Great Gift

Before life, energy worked along physical laws. Once life was created, the plants and animals had to live within these laws. They did not question it. They did not know how. Energy had not endowed them with that ability. They lived in harmony with nature, part of the great energy flow of the Universe. Man's ancestors were also part of that flow, until man developed a logical, analytical side to his thinking (the left side of the brain). It was his great gift, kept in balance with his connection with the Great Spirit, the Energy, with Nature herself. This left side has grown a louder and louder voice as man has developed and evolved. Society has driven this left-sided dominance at the expense of the right-sided intuitive and creative brain. We are trained to listen to the left more than the right side. The ego has become dominant in society, with the quieter and less frequent voice of the right side challenging the *status quo*. Artists, poets, and creative people speak out for the right side of the brain, the intuitive mind, and are trying to show the powers that be that the world needs to be kept in balance. We cannot continue to serve the ego in the manner we have for so long. The left side of the brain uses science, the need for empirical, reproducible evidence, something that can be seen, touched, or dissected. The right side of the brain is happy with feeling, with intuition, or with creativity. There is no need to know *how* it works, only *that* it works.

The right side is not less valid that the left. Nor is the left less valid than the right. They must be in harmony. We need to quiet the left so that we can hear the right. Then the left side will speak when it is important to speak, rather than incessantly chatter like the irritating stranger who will not stop speaking to you on a long coach trip. When we can still the left side, then the wisdom of the right side can flourish. We listen, and so the right side is encouraged to speak more. As it grows, we become aware of its other gifts—the powers of connection, insight, knowing, and understanding that were previously lost to us. We are no longer limited by the knowledge of the left side, but rather open to the wisdom that is available to all.

The Vibrating Universe

All the reactions that I described earlier are part of the dance that is taking place throughout the universe as far as we can tell, creating a powerful energy field that is what the ancient masters might have called "being". If you feel it, it feels alive—although, of course, we know it is not (at least not in the sense of a living, breathing creature). Religious leaders might have called this "being" God. To describe it, man has to call it something, but in fact the best description is for you to feel it.

So what is it that we feel? All things are energy, and energy flows. Energy also vibrates, and this vibration is dependent on the nature of the energy. If it is light energy, then it vibrates along wavelengths that may be visible to the eye. Sounds vibrate enough to affect the ear drum. Light and sound can both vibrate at higher and lower frequencies that humans cannot detect, and man has invented machines to sense these vibrations. Words have specific frequencies that are affected by intonation, pitch, accent, language, and even subject. A serious lecture, a comic improvisation, poetry, or the lyrics to a song all have qualities of vibration that affect our mood, emotion, and feelings. Music has the ability to calm or enrage us, just as words do. Shades of colours have subtle variations that can soothe or agitate us, as can the textures of materials or even materials themselves. Words affect our mood, as do thoughts, each with their own vibration.

Quantum physics describes the universe as a sea of energy and vibration, called the "unified field". This energy condenses into larger and larger objects, from quarks, through to protons and neutrons, which can go on to make atoms that then make molecules—and so it goes on, in ever increasing complexity. Yet, fundamentally all things are the same, built from the same building blocks. According to superstring theory, these building blocks are vibrating elastic loops, and these superstrings are absolutely miniscule (ten million million million times smaller than the nucleus of an atom, it is estimated) vibration tones of this unified field and are the basis of the particles and the forces that make up the universe. As these superstrings coalesce, they create particles, and that is why everything in the universe has a vibration or wave-like nature to it.

A by-product of that vibration is that it sends out ripples into the space around it, and these ripples have energy and corresponding frequencies and vibrations. A hot piece of metal will give off ripples of heat (or electromagnetic radiation) that corresponds to its physical properties. This heat is in turn influenced by the structure of the atoms that make it. The sun radiates great heat due to its immense size and gravity, sending out rays of electromagnetic radiation into the solar system that range from high energy gamma rays to low energy radio waves and everything in between. When matter and waves interact, there is an exchange of energy, the matter is changed, and new waves with new frequencies and vibrations are generated. The entire universe is a jumble of vibrations interacting with each other that help propagate our highly dynamic universe.

Energy and the resulting vibrations are an essential part of our living, dynamic universe, and all things are held together by the fact that heat powers the movement that keeps it connected. Everything gives off some vibration signature, and as we have seen, it is a complex and intricate process. We experience this on a daily basis through the effect music, environments, colours, people, moods, and places have on us. Sounds and images affect the auditory nerve and optic nerve respectively, and both influence the mind and the body through a complex interaction of neurotransmitters, influencing our thoughts, moods, emotions, and physiology.

This creates a stunning complexity that is impossible to visualise and intellectualise. Rather, we feel these vibrations; we can sense them in our bodies. (See the Vibration Exercise later in the book.) As humans we feel the effect of the environment around us, at home, at work, and in the world at large. These vibrations come from many sources—the buildings we are in, the people close to us, the thoughts we have, the tree we sit under, the sun and the moon above, the temperature of the air, the weather, and the time of year. The list is endless, because all things are energy and all energy vibrates and interacts with itself, the unified field. We are aware of interacting with the world in this way. This book simply helps to deepen that awareness, for it is a natural phenomenon that is part of our natural birth right.

The universal vibration of matter may feel more or less uniform throughout the universe; we do not know. The problem with vibrations and waves is that distant ones are easily influenced and overridden by closer ones. The complex vibrations of matter on earth by man must make the universal vibration very difficult to feel. Yet we feel the vibrations of other people and our own vibrations all the time. Animals other than humans, unburdened by the complex emotions we often feel, are in tune with this universal vibration, for they do not have the intellect to generate distorting signals. They live in harmony with the vibrations of planet earth and the universe itself. They are in harmony with themselves and others, in tune with the weather, intuitively aware of the balance of nature, and so they live in harmony with nature. They are rarely ill and have an acceptance of death, because they know it to be the natural way of things.

Man, on the other hand, has his complex thoughts of intellect, jealousy, anger, fear, love, joy, happiness, resentment, regret, and ecstasy to name but a few. Along with deep-seated beliefs, values, and principles, these make the human mind and the environment around that mind a powerful source of distortion. Include in that the minds of all the others you know and share your environment with, and it is a wonder that you can feel anything of the universal vibration at all. Man has created a complex micro-environment around himself that keeps him separate from nature. Radio signals, TV signals, mobile phones, Wi-Fi networks, even the new Cloud technology, are all contributing to the complex wave environment that is influencing the environment around us. Then take into account all the electrical equipment in our homes and work places, each one buzzing and humming and contributing further vibrations into the mix.

The Door to Perception

This is where meditation comes in. As part of the process of going down into meditation, we use breathing to calm and still the mind. This helps to silence so many of the thoughts that send vibrations out and distort the environment around us. Once the mind is calmed, the environment is calmed. Then the still lake is able to receive anything that is there and available for us to receive. Finally, no longer distracted by the day-to-day worries, concerns, thoughts, and feelings we usually have, we can get in touch with something universal that has been there all of the time. We didn't know it was there because we were too busy being confused by other things—things that seemed important at the time and that have consumed our days, weeks, months, and years, until we have had a life time of these thoughts. What if we could still these thoughts, worries, and concerns for a little time every day so that we could listen and feel a vibration that casts these worries and concerns into perspective? Suddenly, we have awareness of a different source of energy and vibration, one that calms us and revitalises us. We allow it to play a significant part in our day, and so it influences us with its calm and beauty. It is the Universe that you feel, and that can only be good.

John Hagelin, PhD, describes meditation like this:

> When our awareness settles, when it withdraws from its sharp outward focus, and this is what meditation is about, meditation turns the attention systematically within, powerfully within, to experience and explore deeper levels of mind, deeper levels of human intelligence. In these deeper levels of mind in this meditative state, more abstract levels of intelligence, correspond to the direct experience of more abstract levels of nature. In the meditative state, the awareness is withdrawn completely and it is expanded maximally, to be abstract, unbounded, universal bliss. In that meditative state our localised awareness has expanded to identify with and become universal awareness. (taken from the interview "The Core of Nature" by John Haglin- interview by Iain McNay. To watch the full interview go to www.conscious.tv)

What wisdom lies there we cannot be sure. What is clear is that whatever wisdom we have manifests itself in thought and even in written or verbal communication. Each thought has a brain wave, which in turn has its own vibration. As we have seen, the universe is full of vibrations, mostly electromagnetic in nature but vibrations nevertheless, which contain wisdom, or rather experience, that can be interpreted by the human mind. It is no coincidence that modern quantum physics is beginning to explain the ideas that ancient masters, mystics, and aesthetics have talked about for thousands of years. It is no wonder that religions have talked about a great creator who has the power to create the heavens and the earth, who is omnipotent and omnipresent, terrible and compassionate, all-knowing and all-seeing.

I am not saying that God is an energy force that vibrates through the universe and communicates through that vibration and that man can interpret these vibrations. But what if that were the case? It makes the wonder of Abraham's and Moses' communication with God just as special and wonderful as it does the revelation to Mohammed or the mission that Joan of Arc was sent upon, the words of Jesus or the conversation between Lord Krishna and Prince Arjuna in the Bhagavad Gita of Hindu scripture. I am not trying to trivialise religion, but rather simply seeking to entwine the evidence of science with the scriptures of religion. It makes it no less wonderful or special in my eyes. In some respects it is more so, for the beauty lies in nature. There is nothing that we need to fear, no God that we must please or appease, simply a universal energy that should be respected and honoured because it gave us life and all the beauty that we see and feel.

Order and Chaos

In short, we come from a very long history of energy that has gone along a journey of change and evolution and that will continue to change and evolve long after the human race has become extinct. We are possibly the first creatures to be able to influence the flow of energy in a conscious way. In the past the energy has flowed in a manner that seemed to be random or chaotic. As we have discussed, this is not the case. There is order within the chaos. Things work too well for it be without order. There are natural laws that energy follows. We are part of that energy, and so we must follow the laws. If we do not follow them, we become crushed by the weight of the power of the energy. If we do follow the laws, we get carried along by the power of the energy, and our lives flow with ease and wonder. This does not mean we will not face hardship and even tragedy, but our life will flow with a vitality and power that makes us feel vital and alive. We have the power to create our future, and our minds are the key to this future. Our minds are designed to work with the energy of the universe. Many books have been published describing methods of achieving this. In essence, by focussing on what we want, we get what we want. It may require a change in thinking, certainly a change in actions, but in time we create the conditions to make things happen. And then they do– spontaneously, naturally, with grace and ease, as if they are falling into your lap. Once we begin to see the intricate manner in which cause and effect work, only then can we truly appreciate the power that the mind has in creating our future. We each play our part, but it cannot be done by us alone. We need the universe on our side. We need to learn to trust it, love it, dance with it, believe in it, and do what we can to help it.

To understand that everything is energy is to realise that we need to be able to work with energy if we want to achieve anything in this lifetime. To help ourselves and to help others requires a strong sense of focus, a channelled energy that is going to make things happen. We must be clear, we must be direct, we must be proud and humble, we must have a voice, and we must listen, for this is all part of the energy flow. Blockages, pain, tiredness, and ill health are signs that the energy is not flowing. We need to seek a different path, find another way, and allow the energy to flow along another path. Life does not have to be difficult. It is in fact easy. We are taught to live in a particular way that is often in contrast to the laws of energy. Our financial crisis, our environmental crisis, our crime crisis, our famine and poverty crises are all signs that everything is not well and that the energy does not flow as it must. We need to find another way, let the energy flow freely, and let it work its magic. In our naivety we have made these mistakes. In our greed we continue to make them. Only in our wisdom can we listen to the energy and work with it and live a life in harmony with nature and energy herself.

Energy is a Big Subject

We all think that we know what energy is. But do we? We turn on a radio or the TV, and it works. We just press a button or turn a knob, and—hey presto—we have power, we have vision, we have colour, and we have sound.

We have these things all of the time around us and in us, but most of us do not acknowledge this. We do not take note of this because it is part of all that makes our lives possible. If we lost our hearing, how difficult would our lives be? If we lost our vision, how difficult would our lives be? We rely on our senses to help us navigate daily life. If we lose any one of our senses, the others seem to take over and compensate for that which we have lost. We absorb and make sense of our external world through our senses and the energy that they send in our direction.

The idea of energy is so simple, and yet it is so difficult to explain. It is that which we take for granted all of the time. Every moment of our lives we have energy coming at us and yet we acknowledge it hardly at all. Why do we not? We do not give the energy a second thought because it is not important to us as long as it is doing for us what it needs to do. It is only when it does not work for us that we really notice it. Our senses make sense of our external environments through the energy that comes at us all of the time. Light is energy, and light is the colour that we see. Sound is energy, and it is what we hear with our ears. Energy is around us all of the time. The wind that rushes past us is energy. The warmth from the sun is energy. A person blowing you a kiss is energy, and the person talking to you is energy, as are their words to you. It is all energy however you look at it. You are energy, I am energy, and the kitchen sink is energy. There is nothing that is not energy.

So why is that important? It is important because at the most fundamental level that is what connects all of us. The fact is everything is energy, and all forms of energy interact with and impact on all other forms of energy. One source of energy can, will, and does affect another source of energy. I am energy, and I now speak to you through my written word. What I am saying to you has energy, it is energy, and you receive it as energy. If I say something to you that upsets you, there will be a response to that from you.

Think of something that someone has said to you in the past that hurt or upset you. Think of that now. Bring it to mind and relive it now. Now how do you feel? Is your heart racing? Do you feel upset? Are you feeling a bit low? Has your mood become depressed? Has it made you cry or brought some tears to your eyes? Are you feeling angry? Have the palms of your hands started to sweat? Are you hot under the collar? These are the types of things that happen to us when we are upset or angry. These are typical responses to another person saying or doing something that has hurt or upset us.

What has really happened to you is this. You have received an energetic encounter with someone, and you have responded to that energetic encounter with energy. If something was said to you, then that is energy. The words are energy, and the words have their own vibration, which is energy in itself. You have felt that energy of the words. They have had resonance upon your physical, mental, and emotional being. You have responded to those words with energy. Your thoughts are energy. They radiate out of your physical body by way of a vibration, and so you send them out into the world and into the situation. The response that your physical body musters as it responds to the hardship of the negative encounter is energy. The heat that the body exudes is energy also. The sweat from the anger is energy. The anger itself is energy. Any sort of action that may come as a result of the negative encounter is energy. We could go on and on, but I am sure you take my point. There is nothing that is not energy. It may come in one form or another, but it is all energy. All that exists is no more than one form of energy or another form of energy. Each form of energy has impact on the other form of energy. We each, a form of energy, are linked to each other as energy.

Interconnection

How simple is that? If we can have impact for the bad then so too we can have impact for the good. I am going to send out a thought right now. Before I do so, I want you to take note of how you are feeling at this very moment. Write it down on a piece of paper: "I feel happy" or "I feel sad" or "I feel like rubbish." Whatever is true for you, write it down. The thought that I am going to send out is this: "I love being alive and living here and now with all that there is." Now say that again to yourself and let it resonate in your being. I sent out a positive thought that is accepting of everything. I have just sent out into the universe a positive thought of acceptance. Everything that thought touches will feel that positivity. It has touched you now. It will have touched you in one way or the other.

Take some time right now to feel in yourself the impact of that thought statement I sent to you and the universe. How do you feel? Do you feel the same as before you read it? Words have power in their meaning. We all know this. The most gifted authors demonstrate to us the power of the written word. Words spoken, written, or thought, have a power in their own vibration. If I think something, I send out to you that thing by way of energy. I send out a vibration, and it is that vibration that is recognised by you. You do not have to hear the meaning. You feel the meaning. Thoughts are subtle energy, and so for most people the interaction that they are having with another person's thoughts passes them by. We have all heard of the aboriginal people of Australia and how they have been reported to be able to communicate with each other through thought. Well, if thought is vibration that is being sent out of the body, then that would indeed be possible. There are also many accounts of mothers who have said they have known that their children have had some form of adversity, and they knew it when it happened. Something told them about it.

I think we are all linked into each other at a vibration level, and we communicate with each other all of the time by sending out vibrations to each other. We exude energy all of the time, and each of us reads this energy that is being sent in our direction. We *feel* each other. I also think that the more we are connected emotionally, the stronger the vibration connection is between us. So therefore we have a stronger connection to those people who love us or know us well, like close family and friends. I had a very beautiful friend many years ago. This lady has now sadly passed away. When we were young women, I very often would call at her house, usually on my way to or from work. I did shift work in those days, and my friend lived en route to my job. When I would turn up at her door, more often than not she would say to me, "I knew you were coming today; I thought about you." Or she would say that she knew I would bring this or that today. This sort of thing happened all of the time between us. The knowing would be on both sides. I know that there are many of you reading this who will know just what I am talking about, as it happens to you all of the time with some people more than others.

We are all connected on an energetic level and on a vibration level also. This is why this sort of thing happens to so many of us all of the time. If you say this does not happen to you, I feel it does happen in some way or other, but you just do not listen to what is given to you. These vibration messages are subtle, they are quiet, and we have to learn to hear them. We each have to learn to listen and to trust what is coming in our direction if they are to be truly useful to us. Of course they will be useful however we receive them, for even if we do not know on a conscious level that we are receiving them and we receive them purely subconsciously, we are still none the less receiving them. Our subconscious will register the information, and it will still therefore be at our disposal.

Energy Manipulation

So now you understand that you are interconnected on an energetic and vibration level, now what? How does that affect you one way or the other? Well, to be honest, it makes no real difference to your life. If you did not understand this, life would trundle on for you just the same, no difference. However, the knowing and understanding of this gives you power. It gives you the power to choose how you use it. You could further explore this concept and learn how to tap into the ability and strengthen and develop it. If you could develop the ability to hear people's thoughts, how would that affect your life? If you could develop the ability to connect to others, how would that affect your life? What could you do with that knowledge and ability? I cannot promise that you will be able to walk down any street and hear passing persons' thoughts. However, with time and practise you will most certainly be in better tune with other people, and who knows how far this knowledge and ability can take you?

What we are talking about here is developing the ability to connect into another person on an energetic level and to feel the vibration and the messages within those energetic waves that they are sending out into the wider world. The wind can be subtle or aggressive, and so too can the energy that I speak of here. It takes time to find it within oneself. There are exercises that can be done to strengthen one's ability to find the energy that exists within. Anyone can at will pull this energy into their body. It is like anything else; it just needs some knowledge and a bit of know-how. If you are willing to be open-minded and give a little of your time, then within the pages of this book you will find the knowledge to help you find your own personal energy.

Energy Manipulation Exercise to Help Sense Energy

To help you start to feel the energy that I have been talking about, there are many exercises to bring this about. This is one that was taught to me and one that I use when teaching my students.

Bringing Energy down into the Body

1. Imagine there is a ball of white light energy above your head (a ball of sun light to you and me).

2. Now with the power of the imagination bring that energy down through the crown of the head slowly into the body.

3. Now in steps and stages bring the white light energy (sunlight) down into the body to the solar plexus (upper tummy, just under the bust) area.

4. Now allow the energy to sit there in the solar plexus for a while.

5. Now with your imagination grow the energy in the solar plexus so that it grows from the size of a tennis ball to a beach ball.

6. When you feel that you have a large ball of energy, send this energy out from the solar plexus into the room.

We can make energy move in and out of our bodies with the power of the mind. You may feel that you have done nothing at all and feel that you did not move energy into and out of your body. This is normal when we first do this exercise. As you practise this exercise more and more, the feeling of energy moving into the body and out of the body will grow. You will become more sensitive to feeling the energy moving through your body.

Energy moves through our body all the time, but most people are just not consciously aware of it. Some people are very sensitive to this movement of energy and can manipulate it at will.

There are many purposes to this exercise. If I were teaching a person to feel other people's energy very strongly, I would give them this exercise to do regularly to strengthen their ability to sense energy within their own bodies first.

There is a second part to this exercise, and that is to send the energy in a deliberate direction. Do you have a willing friend who will help you with this? It is best if you do not know this person too well. The less you know about this person, the better. So you need to find a person who you know reasonably well and who will be a good sport to allow you to try this on them.

Now send the energy in their direction by imagining the energy being sent from your solar plexus to their solar plexus. Now pull the energy back to yourself. Ask yourself these questions: "What do I feel about this person?" and "How does this person make me feel?" (not "What do I think about this person?"– they are two entirely different things).

So what is the answer? How does this person make you feel? What do you feel about this person? What do you feel that you know about this person? Practice this exercise on as many people as you can.

Your ability to feel energy in general and the energy of others in particular will improve dramatically. In time you will know things about people and their lives that logically you should not know. In time your accuracy will improve, and eventually you will become one hundred per cent spot on with the information that you will be able to deduce about others.

How interesting is that?

Waves Creating the Future

Nothing happens instantly. There is an illusion of instantaneous action or reaction, but in truth nothing is instantaneous. All action requires thought in attitude, in perspective, in belief, and in values. All actions are the result of some thought, so there is always a delay between thought and action.

The time of that delay is what confuses us. An athlete wins a competition. This is the result of many years' work, many thoughts piling up into a tidal wave of the future, a tidal wave of energy that creates so much momentum that it creates a champion. Enough waves of the right frequency pile up to create such a big wave that it creates a champion. *It takes consistently directed, constant thoughts towards a given goal to allow us to direct our future.* Powerful thoughts become the force that overcomes all obstacles in our path. So strong a force does not produce instant results. It takes time for the ripples to build up, and they can only build up in the future, ahead of you. They travel ahead of you, building your future potential, and you catch up.

Ripple upon ripple upon ripple, and your future is set by you so far ahead of the present that you do not see how it can work. No champion becomes a champion without the work being put in for years before. No great actor or musician has not had years of anonymity without success. They burst onto the scene, but that is not the beginning of their journey; it is the start of your awareness. An athlete puts in years of hard work to be number one. This is all part of The Way or The Path. If it was an instant thing, it would be called *The Step*. Dedication, perseverance, patience, and a belief that you are moving towards a goal allow you to feel yourself growing. It is the increase of momentum that enables you to feel the *greater you* evolving. It is inevitable.

All this does not happen without the work beforehand. Fleeting thoughts and pipe dreams cannot result in success. There is not the sustained pressure of thought to create a reality. Reality requires more than that. It requires a wave—a tidal wave. That is why habits are so hard to break. You must change your thoughts consistently, and in so doing, you change the nature of the wave of the future. This is the hardest part. You give up too soon. Just as the nature of the wave starts to change significantly, so you change your thoughts back, and the nature of the future wave resumes its old form. It is at this time that you must have the deepest resolve. Understand the process that you can win out, and soon, very soon, you will be walking a different path. You started weeks ago, but only now are you reaping the benefit of your hard work.

New scenery, new friends, a new job, and new future—whatever it is, it is the result of your past thoughts. Whatever is happening in your life now is because of your past thoughts. Much of what you do, particularly much of how you react, is based on past thoughts. A new perspective creates different thoughts. It may happen quickly, but it is not instantaneous.

Thought- action

Action- reaction

In our wisdom, we cannot truly know where our thoughts will lead us. There are too many variables. We are not isolated, and there are so many other people with their thoughts and their waves interacting with ours that we cannot know the outcome. Life throws left-field balls we just did not see. In time we learn not to become so attached to what we want. We learn to plan, hedge our bets, scheme, and manipulate, but we must understand that we are not totally in control.

We can learn to play the game. Play it and become a master at it! There is no greater game, and there is no greater achievement. Success is dependent on understanding this equation. The balance of all things at all times, the infinite variability of universal forces.

The only place where success comes before work is in a dictionary.

—Vidal Sassoon

Growth Comes Slowly

Growth comes slowly.

Faith is easily knocked,

But we must have faith,

And we must have patience.

Only with faith and patience

Can we hope to achieve our goals and dreams,

Fulfil our potential, and find the horizon we seek.

I write to set things in motion.

I write to increase momentum,

Until change becomes the truth,

And truth becomes reality.

David Brown

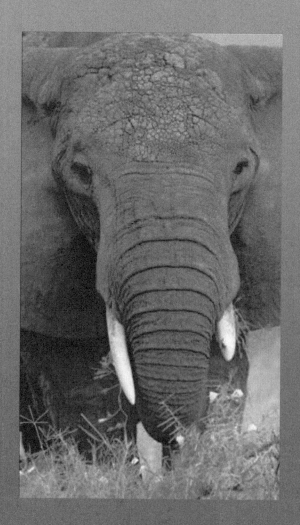

Vibration

Everything in the universe vibrates. All things are held together by the rate at which the quantum soup vibrates. Everything in the universe is not always what it seems to us. We seem solid, and most matter seems solid to us, but nothing is solid. All things that exist are mostly made up of space and are being held together by vibration.

We all feel this vibration of matter, because we are connected to it. We ourselves are matter, and we vibrate as all things do. Each thing and person has a different quality of vibration. It is almost as though each thing has its own vibration signature. We can differentiate one thing from the other by the quality and feel of the vibration it is emitting. The vibrations in all things are very subtle, and some people feel the different vibrations very acutely once they concentrate on them. Other people feel the vibrations very slightly and have to concentrate hard on each particular vibration to feel it. These people usually need to do the vibration exercise many times before the full effect of the exercise is felt and understood. Some people are super-sensitive to the vibrations, and other people are less so.

People have their own vibrations, and we can know each person by their vibration. People have many attributes by which we can identify them. People have a sound to them by way of their voice, and this is a vibration because sound is vibration. People have their own personal physical smell, and this too is a vibration because smell is a vibration. People have their own colour and colouring, for example, hair, eye, and skin colouring. Colour is also a vibration, because colour is light and light is a vibration. Although these vibrations are easy to understand and we all know them, these are not the vibrations that I am talking about here. There is another vibration that we have that is to do with our mass holding together. If we did not vibrate, we would disintegrate and be a pile of formless matter on the floor. We would be just a pile of dust.

I have a good friend who is a professional medium. Some years ago when we were both developing as mediums, there was an interesting incident that I would like to share with you. My friend used to say to me that all people have their own buzz to them. She was talking about the vibration that I am trying to explain here. I did not know in those days what she was talking about. I listened to her, as she knew more than I did in those days about the mechanics of mediumship and she would tell me many things.

My friend and I would go to a coffee shop after class with many of our friends from class. One particular day my friend seemed a little up in the air, so to speak. She was not calm, and she was a little frazzled. There had been a student who had once attended our class whom my friend had not liked too much. This lady and my friend seemed to clash. As we approached the coffee shop my friend became more agitated, and when we enquired what the matter was, my friend replied that this lady whom my friend did not like was in the vicinity. When we asked her where, my friend replied that she did not know, but she could feel and hear her buzz. As we all sat down for coffee and snacks, my friend became more and more unsettled.

My friend eventually said that the lady was in the shop across the road. We could not see her, and we had not seen any one walk past us. I was facing the shop and had not seen the person in question. Our other friends and I were not inclined to believe my friend, as we had not seen this woman, and we would have done so because the street was not a busy one. All afternoon we were in the coffee shop, as was our custom each week. My friend kept saying, "She is there in that shop across the street." The shop that my friend pointed to was an odd shop, and we could not ascertain from the frontage what sort of shop it was. During the course of the afternoon my fellow classmates drifted off home one by one, and eventually there were just three of us left—my friend, myself, and one other class member. Well, as soon as the majority of the class had disappeared, the woman that my friend had said was in the shop came out. The other lady and I were in disbelief. We just could not believe it. There she was as my friend had said. When I asked my friend how she knew, she replied, "I would know that buzz anywhere." My friend's senses are supersensitive.

It would be ridiculous for me to say to you that you will have the same sensitivity as my friend. You possibly will not, although of course there will be some people who will. We all have varying abilities in all things, and just because one person can do something easily does not mean that all people can. By the same token, it does not mean either that no one else will be able to do the same or similar. It is a matter of trying the exercise and finding out where you are with your own sensitivity to vibration.

As with all exercises of this nature that are developing sensitivity, the more you do them, the better you will become. The purpose of this exercise is to help you tap into something that already exists within you. It is to help you do so consciously and methodically.

I was taught this vibration exercise by my teacher Janette Marshall. This is her exercise, and she has kindly allowed us to use it here for you to experience. When I did this exercise with Janette for the first time, I felt each vibration distinctly, clearly, and profoundly. This was an eye-opening exercise for me. I have done this exercise many times with many of my own students, and each student has a different reaction to the experience of doing this exercise. Some, like me, are blown away with what they feel, whilst others say, "What vibration?" Still others say, "Umm, I did feel some things but not others." Every person is different and experiences this exercise differently. Everything has a vibration; each thought, feeling, idea, and physical thing will give a vibration within us.

The Vibration Exercise

To do the exercise you will need to have a friend to help you. One of you will do the exercise, and the other will read out the instructions. The person doing the exercise needs to stand up and close their eyes. The person reading the instructions can sit down if they choose to do so.

Your friend needs to say:

1. Stand still and close your eyes.

2. Relax and take some deep breaths.

3. Now listen to my instructions.

4. I would like you to take your awareness to your body. I would like you to feel your body with your awareness.

5. How does it feel to you? Are there any aches and pains, or is it totally relaxed? Understand how your body feels. Take a moment to do this.

6. Now I would like you to feel the vibration of your own body. To do this say in your mind "I would like to feel the vibration of my own body" and then relax and just feel what comes back to you. Relax first, and now say, "I wish to feel the vibration of my own body." Know that what you feel is the vibration of your own body.

7. Now I would like you to take your awareness outside of yourself and I would like you to say to yourself, "I would like to feel the vibration of the universe".
    Now just take a moment to feel that.

8. Now I would like you to feel the vibration of the concept, the Earth.
    Now just take a moment to feel that.

9. Now I would like you to feel the vibration of the concept, Mother.
    Now just take a moment to feel that.

10. Now I would like you to feel the vibration of the concept, Father.
    Now just take a moment to feel that.

11. Now I would like you to feel the vibration of the concept, Brother.
    Now just take a moment to feel that.

12. Now I would like you to feel the vibration of the concept, Sister.
    Now just take a moment to feel that.

13. Now I would like you to feel the vibration of the concept, Friend.
    Now just take a moment to feel that.

14. Now I would like you to feel the vibration of the concept, Enemy.
    Now just take a moment to feel that.

15. Now I would like you to feel the vibration of the concept, Happiness.
    Now just take a moment to feel that.

16. Now I would like you to feel the vibration of the concept, Sadness.
    Now just take a moment to feel that.

17. Now I would like you to feel the vibration of the concept, Tranquillity.
    Now just take a moment to feel that.

18. Now I would like you to feel the vibration of the concept, Disturbance.
    Now just take a moment to feel that.

19. Now I would like you to feel the vibration of the concept, Danger.
    Now just take a moment to feel that.

20. Now I would like you to feel the vibration of the concept, War.
    Now just take a moment to feel that.

21. Now I would like you to feel the vibration of the concept, Living.
    Now just take a moment to feel that

22. Now I would like you to feel the vibration of the concept, Death.
    Now just take a moment to feel that.

23. Now I would like you to feel the vibration of the concept, Anger.
    Now just take a moment to feel that.

24. Now I would like you to feel the vibration of the concept, Joy.
    Now just take a moment to feel that.

25. Now I would like you to feel the vibration of the concept, Arrogance.
    Now just take a moment to feel that.

26. Now I would like you to feel the vibration of the concept, Subservience.
    Now just take a moment to feel that.

27. Now I would like you to feel the vibration of the concept, Violence.
    Now just take a moment to feel that.

28. Now I would like you to feel the vibration of the concept, Fun.
    Now just take a moment to feel that.

29. Now I would like you to feel the vibration of the concept, Laughter.
    Now just take a moment to feel that.

30. Now I would like you to feel the vibration of the concept, Noise.
    Now just take a moment to feel that.

31. Now I would like you to feel the vibration of the concept, Quiet.
    Now just take a moment to feel that.

32. Now I would like you to feel the vibration of the concept, Struggle.
    Now just take a moment to feel that.

33. Now I would like you to feel the vibration of the concept, Ease.
    Now just take a moment to feel that.

34. Now I would like you to feel the vibration of the concept, Peace.
    Now just take a moment to feel that.

35. Now I would like you to feel the vibration of the concept, Balance.
    Now just take a moment to feel that.

It is better if there is not a long time between each concept. Just a minute would be sufficient to feel each one. You could add to this list and see what you feel with each new thing added.

The principal aim of the Eastern mystical traditions is . . . .

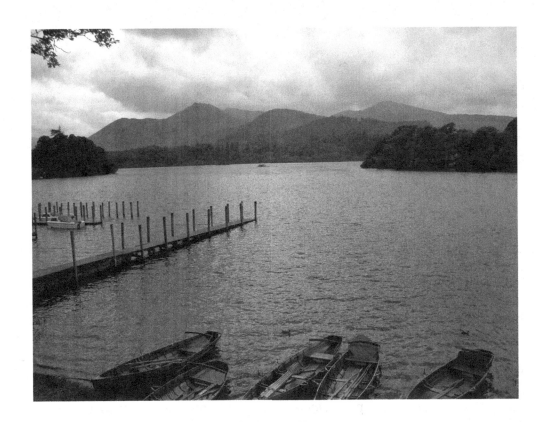

...therefore to readjust the mind by centring and quietening it through meditation. The Sanskrit term for meditation—Samadhi—means literally "mental equilibrium". It refers to the balanced and tranquil state of mind in which the basic unity of the Universe is experienced"

—Fritjof Capra

Entering into the Samadhi of purity, [one obtains] all penetrating insight that enables one to become conscious of the absolute oneness of the Universe.

— Ashvaghosha

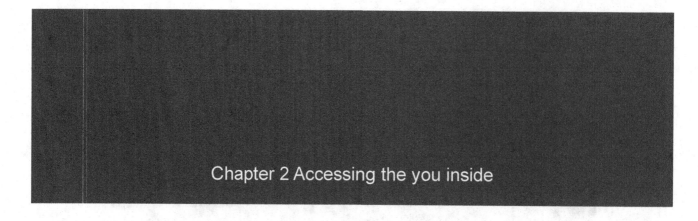

Accessing You

This is the chapter that I have feared writing the most. Maybe I should have left it until the end of writing the book. However, here I am diving right on in. Why is this chapter so hard for me to write? I have agonised about how to start this chapter. This book is called *Nourish the Flame Within*, and this chapter is called "Accessing the "You Inside". Some people who are reading this now will understand straight away what those two titles mean. Others reading this will wonder what on earth we are trying to share. In fact, "share" is a good word. The word "share" means to give part of something you have to someone else. We do have something we wish to share with you. This book has been written with the intention that what we wish to share with you should take you on a journey through your life. This book can be used as a tool to help you in many ways in your life. It is the intention of this book that all of the information provided should be a complete whole, and this chapter gives you solid ground to build your life on. Indeed, all of the chapters are tools that you the reader can use in any way you choose. It may be that you will only use one part of the book, or you might use the entire book. You can start at the beginning if you wish and go through it end to end. Or you can just dive in anywhere that suits you best and take what you will from wherever you choose within the book. It is your choice. What works best for you is what is best for you.

The meditations in this book are a tool to help strengthen each area of your life. We are not suggesting that you or your life happen to be weak. However, each one of us in life, no matter who we happen to be—whether we are high-born or low-born—will encounter some form of difficulty or misfortune in some measure at some point during our life. If you have the good fortune to be young and at the very beginning of your life, it may well be your belief that what we say to you here is nonsense. What we would say to you in that case is go and find a person who has life etched on their brow and ask them this question: "Have you managed to live your life without any hurt, difficulty, or harm coming your way?" The older the person you ask, the less likely the person will be to have lived their life without struggle having befallen them. For it is through the difficulties of our lives that we gain the most out of our lives. It is the difficulties that teach us strength, patience, pain, loss, loneliness, happiness, sadness, self-resilience, self-reliance, co-operation, communication, self-awareness and love, to name but a handful of things. We learn so much about our world, ourselves, and other people through the difficult experiences that come our way during our lives.

We have to make a response to every situation that comes our way. We have choice in each of those situations. In fact, sometimes there are too many choices, while at other times we feel we have no choice at all.

Whatever we choose to do in any situation will indeed have impact on our lives, our emotions, and our relationships. Sometimes at our lowest points in life we may well feel alone. We may well feel that the world has turned against us and we have nowhere to be and nowhere to turn. The truth is that you are never alone. You only have to look around you to know that separation and the feeling of aloneness is just a temporary illusion. The illusion is temporary, because if you wish to let the illusion go and pass it out to the Universe, it will indeed float away. In reality, being alone is merely a thought—a thought that you are having at this point in time, one that you are in fact in control of. Take a look outside of your home. Amongst the houses and the cars, what do you see there? People, my friend, are all around you. There are billions of people sharing this life with you. Each one of those people is a soul to be connected with. If you give them the time and opportunity to know you, then you will have people in your life. It takes time to make those connections, but friendships are forged that way. Time, love, kindness, and offering the hand of true friendship are the keys here, my friend.

There is another aspect to this idea of being alone or not alone. The first three meditations in this book give us some insight into that connection which I just spoke to you about. Here we come to the difficult part of this chapter. Just as we spoke of the interconnection of things in the science chapter, so there is a reality far beyond you. There is a reality that exists outside of you. Take a look up at the night sky and look at the stars. What do you think is out there? We each have our own idea of what lies beyond this life and this beautiful earth that we all share. Close your eyes and picture the stars. This is the stuff that you are made of. The stars are energy, and so are you. You have a connection to them, and they have one to you. Yet they are so far from you! How could they be connected to you? A tree is far removed from you, and yet it is closer to you.

Perhaps proximity is not the key. Perhaps the stuff of life and the essence of life are the key. All things are energy, and there is a relationship between all things and you. You are connected at a fundamental level to all that there is and all that there ever will be. You live and you die. You are here and then you are gone from this life. People ask how we can know that there is life after life. How can we be sure? Close your eyes and be quiet for a time. Sit in a place and just be. Sit in a place that is free from noise—a field, a quiet room, anywhere noise free and people-free. Now just give yourself some time to be you. Take your shoes off and feel the earth beneath your feet. Just stand in bare feet on any water-soaked beach and feel it. In fact, go the whole hog. Lay flat starfish style on that water-soaked beach, close your eyes, and just stay there for a time. Do nothing, say nothing; *feel everything*. What is it that you are feeling? What is it that you are sensing? Do you feel anything at all? Do you feel everything that there is to feel? Who are you and what are you? What is life about, and how do you connect to it?

For some of you reading this, all of these questions and impressions that I have given here will resonate at a deep and fundamental level, but I can hear others saying, "What is that woman talking about?" Or there will be words to that effect. To be fair, if you are reading this book, if you have this book and have opened its pages, there must be a part of you that feels some of these ideas and questions. There must be a part of you that yearns for the answers.

There must in some part of your being be a feeling that there is indeed more to this life than the popular social view. This popular social view goes something like this. We are born to parents we did not choose and who did not choose us. We are sent to be schooled mostly against our will, and we are taught a whole array of things that we are told will benefit us. However, we mostly cannot see how, when, or where that benefit will come. We go along with the idea because we are children and have no power or choice. We are trained for work, and we mostly end up in jobs we hate. Or if we do not actively hate our jobs, we just accept our fate, get on with it and comply with what we have come to understand as being true for us. We have friends who have mostly drifted into our lives as we have theirs. We walk through life in a powerless and chaotic fashion with mostly no direction and with no real choice on our part. We are individuals who are connected to a few. We are connected to a few of the human race directly by blood, but as for the rest of life on earth, it is there to be exploited and used at will. When we die, that is it—a welcome and final end to a life of misery, toil, blandness, and apathy.

We Say . . .

Of course not everyone views life like that. Of course, there are the lucky few who have it all—the lifestyle, the notoriety, the glitz, and the glamour—and, of course, if only you were they and they were you! If only you were born to their parents or had their looks, their brains, or their opportunity. Life would have been so much better and so completely different. A better life and a better you— those are the things that most people want.

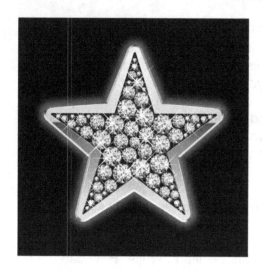

It is one view of life to view others as" having it all". However, material wealth and glitz and glamour are the superficial trappings of life. They are the trappings to which we are too often programmed to aspire. The things that last and are real are the things that one cannot buy.

We are who we are in this moment in time, and that person is a product of what has passed before in our lives. It does not matter to whom we were born or where we grew up. It comes down to being as true to yourself as you can be. To fulfil your uniqueness, you can only be you.

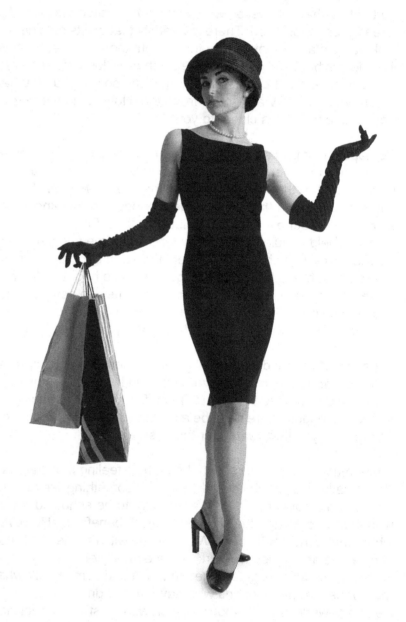

Of course not everyone views life like that. Of course, there are the lucky few who have it all—the lifestyle, the notoriety, the glitz, and the glamour—and, of course, if only you were they and they were you! If only you were born to their parents or had their looks, their brains, or their opportunity. Life would have been so much better and so completely different. A better life and a better you—those are the things that most people want. The trouble is, we only have ourselves in the here and the now. That is it, and that is what you have to work with.

I have to say there have been times in my life when I have wondered what this life we have all been born into is all about. Did we ask to be here? Or is it all random, and are we just here by chance? These questions are real and valid. Of course, since we have all found ourselves here in this life, it is our right to wonder and suppose—to wonder to what is the purpose of life itself and to suppose the answer to that question also.

This book is not about religion. Many people throw the words "spiritual" and "spirituality" around as they would throw a designer scarf over their shoulder. They either wear them as objects or hide from them as if they were rude words. "Spirit" and "spiritual" are neither of those things. At your core you are spirit. You are a spiritual being. It is not something you need to learn or need to become. You are it. You do not even have to acknowledge you are it. You are spiritual whether you wish to be or not. Just as you are a "human", so too you are a "spirit". Being a spiritual being does not depend on your thought or your action or anything you may or may not learn. You are spirit from the moment you are born to the moment you die. It is my personal belief that life continues far beyond this life and that we do not die but rather just change existence. That is my personal belief. I am sure you have yours. Whatever your personal belief is, that is fine. What is right for you, is right. For we each need to make sense of this life in our own way. We need to have that which sits comfortably with us. For, wherever you are at this moment in your beliefs and understandings, that is the right place for you to be. Other people may have different understandings to you, and that is right for them.

We are not static beings. We are beings that learn and grow, and our understanding of life grows as we grow. Everything we do and take on board within our understanding changes us for all time. We can never go back to who we were; we must sit with who we are now. We can only accept who other people are for who they are now and rejoice in that. These first three meditations are there to help you connect and develop as a spiritual being. You may understand what I am talking about, or you may not. It does not matter one bit where you are or even where you want to be. If you do these three meditations regularly, you will connect to spirit. You will find your inner self. You will find the connection that you have to all that there is in the Universe. At a fundamental level we are all connected. We are all energy and we are all human and we are all spirit. These meditations are there for those people who wish to explore that part of their being.

The spirit part of us is us. Our body is the house that we inhabit whilst we are on the earth. It enables us to live this life in this way. I personally have never felt that I am my body. You may agree with what I am saying here or you may not. It is no matter. It does not matter which is true for you. The meditations will have a fundamental impact on you. On a physical level they will help you to feel better. They will help with emotional strength and will have a physical effect in improving your health to a greater or lesser degree. Meditation on a regular basis has been proven to be beneficial in many illnesses and is known to be good for us, just as taking regular exercise is good for us. These meditations throughout the book will help you, your life, your body, your emotional state, and you the spirit person. They will help you connect with you the spirit person like a voyage of rediscovery. Do them regularly and correctly, and they will change you for the better. Who does not what to be a better them? We all do. We all want to be the best us possible.

We Say . . .

Let us try to define "spirit" and "spiritual" in a way that is less emotive. "Spiritual" is so often considered the remit of religion. But what if our earlier description of the universe—that the universe has been built by evolving energy developing through generations of change—is the basis of our spiritual experience? That "spirit" is that energy and that "spiritual" is what we experience or feel when we are connected to that energy? Then, if you are religious, you would call that energy "god", and if you were not religious, you can still think of that spiritual experience without mixing it with religion.

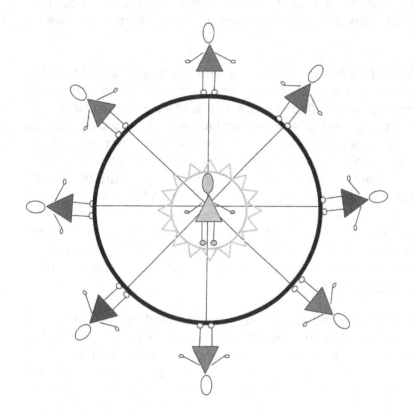

Maybe a way of looking at the issue of religion is to think of the energy of God sitting at the heart of the Universe and to imagine that we are all connected to that energy through energy. Maybe we could also say that we are all trying to both define that energy with our intellect and also perfect the small part of that energy that we ourselves are. We in our own personal ways are trying to become more like that perfect energy. Therefore we could say that science and all religions and also those who have no religion all are on their personal road to God.

We Say . . .

Pain and hardship are written into life, just as joy and wonderment are. Through life's experience we can learn to turn stumbling blocks into stepping stones. For it is through the difficulties of our lives that we gain the most learning. It is the difficulties that teach us strength, patience, pain, loss, loneliness, happiness, sadness, self-resilience, self-reliance, co-operation, communication, self-awareness, and love to name but a handful of things.

We can learn so much about our world and ourselves and other people through the difficult experiences that come our way during our lives. In every situation that comes our way, we have to make a response to it. We have choice in each of these situations. In fact, sometimes there are too many choices, while at other times we feel we have no choice at all.

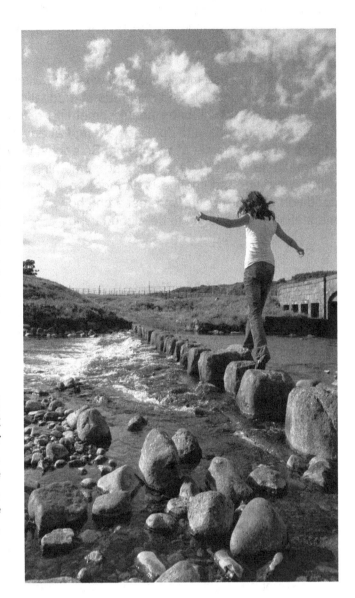

Meditation

When many people first decide to try meditation, they come up against their first stumbling block. How do I do it? The next set of questions will be: "What is it? What am I meant to be doing and achieving from it? Do I need to take all thoughts out of my mind whilst I do it? If I do, then how do I do that?"

The first thing I need to tell you is to relax. Relaxation is an important part of meditation. The next thing I need to tell you is not to worry about what you should or should not be doing; all will become clear if you follow the steps as I explain them to you. Meditation is such a useful and beautiful practice. Once you understand what can be achieved in meditation, there will be no going back. It will always be part of your life. I am not saying that you will do it on a daily basis or that when you meditate you will do so for a certain amount of time each time you meditate. In fact, that is not the approach to meditation that I would recommend to you, because that is making it a chore. It should not be a chore but something that you return to as and when you need it. It is a tool for enhancing yourself, your selfawareness, and the quality of your health and your life. Meditation is a tool, and that is all. Once you learn how to do it, you will have the ability to meditate for life. Meditation can refresh and revive you. It can take you deep into yourself and change your self-awareness. It can connect you to a reality beyond this one and on to truly beautiful things.

How you wish to use meditation and what you wish to gain from it will depend on what meditation you do. There are hundreds and hundreds of meditations, all with different purposes. Each meditation that you choose to do will bring about something different within you, depending on the purpose of the meditation you choose to do. Each attempt at any meditation will bring about some change within you on one level or another of your being. So each time you meditate it will be different, because each time you meditate you will have changed something within yourself. You will have developed something within yourself, and change is change, so there is no returning to the old you. You can change the condition of your health, and research shows this is the truth. We can enhance our overall health by meditating. That has got to be a good thing!

The Purpose of Meditation

There is an overall purpose to meditation, which is to bring calm and balance to the body. If our body is calm and balanced, we are more likely to be healthy, as we are reducing as far as we can stress of all kinds within the body. Meditation is really a very deep relaxation, and it takes a little practise to learn. Once learnt, meditation will help us to help ourselves achieve that overall purpose.

Along with calmness and balance meditation has three other purposes. We can say that the following are the four main purposes:

1. To bring calm and balance to the mind and body

2. To connect the person to their spiritual selves

3. To connect the person to a spiritual reality beyond themselves

4. To bring about a realisation of truth, understanding, and awareness

The first purpose is to bring about calm to the mind and body. Current thinking and research into meditation is of the opinion that meditation can have significant health benefits. There has been a great deal of research done into the health benefits of meditation since the 1960s, and that research has indicated that it can have a significant impact on many areas of our physical and psychological well-being. Of course, there are too many people who remain sceptical of the documented research, and for those people perhaps no amount of proof will be enough. However, it is my opinion that it makes sense to keep ourselves in a state of calm throughout our day and throughout our lives in general. I can personally see no benefit to being a stressed-out mess on a daily basis. Just those words alone conjure up a powerful image of a person who is out of control and heading for a disaster of one kind or another healthwise.

We have all met such people, I am sure, and in my experience they are the people who find their way eventually to the doctor's surgery looking for help with sleep, heart conditions, stress, etc. If I look back at some of the people in my family who became severely ill, I would say that there is a relationship between their lack of calm due to life's stresses and their sudden ill health. I cannot prove that; it is only my own observation and opinion. Speaking for myself and my own ill health that I suffered years ago, I know deep within my own being that this is the case. I was a stressed-out mess for more years than I can remember. I rushed here and rushed there, attending to everyone else but myself. My work, my study, my husband, my home, my children, my broader family, and everything else came before my own well-being. My body just eventually said "enough", and I found myself with first a viral infection, followed by ME (myalgic encephalomyelitis)for many years. How many women or people in general are reading this now and are thinking, "Oops, that sounds just like me." Whether you believe the research into meditation or not, it is my personal opinion that anything that can help us come to a place of calm has to be a good thing, if only to help us reduce the stress we place on ourselves daily. Meditation is not a cure-all practise. It does not replace your GP. One should be mindful of going for regular medical check-ups. However, meditation can help you to take control of your own health and well-being by creating some positive input rather than the thoughtless negatives that so many of us put into our daily lives. In the past, unfortunately, I could include myself in that group.

The second purpose of meditation is to connect you the physical you, to yourself. What a strange thing to say. "To connect you to you", however, it is not really so strange. It is a bit like taking time to smell the roses. We have such busy lives. We rush here and we rush there, and so often there is little time or opportunity to just be with ourselves and our own thoughts. So what I am saying is that there are two yous. The first is your body and the second is the inner you. Some people think of this as your spirit or your soul or just your inner thoughts or the observer you. However you wish to think of that "you" is fine. All we need to do is to enable you to find it. That bit of you is so often left and forgotten amidst life's rush. We wish to help you nurture that bit of you, bring it back into your life, and not allow it to be side lined and forgotten. That bit of you deserves to be cared about, as it is the best bit of you. It is the bit of you that is who you really are.

The third purpose on our list is to connect the person to a reality beyond this one. Well, we all know that spiritual people have sought this ability long and hard. For thousands of years spiritual people have retreated from ordinary daily life in search of this truth and reality. They have often set aside all that material life has to offer in search and contemplation of something higher, something beyond the daily humdrum that mere mortals have to endure. What was it that these people sought, and, more to the point, did they ever find it? Well, meditation has the ability to take the ordinary and make it extraordinary. That is the best I can tell you or explain to you. In the type of meditation that is designed to expand your awareness, you will indeed find gold—not the metal itself, but something much, much, more, something that is infinitely more useful to you and thus much better. You will find a place that you can retreat to when you need to go there. Each of us has our own levels of tolerances to the stresses of daily life. Sometimes we reach a place that is truly bleak, and we feel that there is no return from that place. There *is* a return. It is merely that you have not yet learnt certain truths about life and do not know the places to find the answers to the difficulties that may be engulfing your person or your life at any particular time. We all seek truth and reality in one way or another. Unfortunately, we do not all find it. However, it is the purpose of this book to help you learn to find it.

The first meditations in this book, which are at the end of this chapter, are designed to help anyone who wishes to find that deeper truth about life to walk the necessary path to that place. If you do the first three meditations regularly, you will speed up the journey to spiritual wisdom and understanding by allowing yourself the connection to that spiritual reality beyond yourself. Once you gain that connection or—should I say?—regain that connection, it will be a part of you forever. You will know where you need to go and how to get there and what is there once you arrive.

The last purpose on our list is truth, understanding, and awareness. "The truth of what?" I hear you ask! What is life about? Why am I here? What is my purpose within life itself? These are weighty questions. I often used to hear my mother say when I was a little girl, "What is it all about? Why are we all going through this?" I think that really what she was asking was, "What is life about?" In her times of strife those would be her musings. I am sure many of us have been at that point often enough, confused and perplexed at what life is serving up for us at that moment. So if we manage to find the answers to life and the truth of what life is about, then we indeed have understanding and awareness as they will follow knowledge.

How to Meditate

Before we begin to meditate, we have to learn how to take ourselves down into relaxation. For this we need to use the power of the breath. By taking slow and deep breaths, we alter our brainwave patterning, and this takes us into an altered state of awareness. By breathing slowly and deeply, we relax the mind and body and thus allow connection to our own spirit or that of the Universe.

We all alter our states of awareness each and every day. We have all done something like driving or walking where we have just not taken note of the journey and wondered where we were for part of the journey. We were oblivious as we did it. We were on autopilot, and this is the sort of state that we need to achieve for meditation. (We do not recommend that you meditate whilst driving, as there are obvious dangers to that. We are just illustrating a point here.)

It is not difficult to achieve this altered state. It may seem a little strange at first as we try to achieve this state. However, the more we practise, like anything else the better we become at it. It is not natural for us to let go of ourselves, but this is what we need to do to achieve meditation. It is a letting go of our conscious awareness or the awake and alert us.

The breath pattern is important for achieving meditation. The important thing to know about the breath is that it should be slow and deep. Ensuring that your breath is both slow and deep will take you down into a meditative state very quickly. It will do so without any further help from you. It is commonly thought by many people that to meditate there has to be a long and arduous road of learning how to do it. This is not so. A minimum amount of time and a little practise will ensure you become a master at meditation.

It is also commonly thought that one has to empty the mind in meditation. For certain types of meditation this may well be the case. For the meditation practice that we are instructing within the confines of this book it is not the case. By using the power of the breath, you will achieve a true meditative state very easily. There is nothing much to it. I would love to say that you need to do this or that or the rest, but that is not the truth of what you need to do. The key is the breath pattern that will take you where you need to be. It is very easy and simple and truly powerful. In the meditative state the body can do remarkable things. It can help itself to heal. It can refresh and renew itself. It can allow the spirit part of the self to travel outside of the physical body to another reality. It can also allow other spiritual beings to connect to it on a spiritual level. All of these things and more are possible in a meditative state. You are always in control in meditation. You can bring yourself back to the here and now whenever you choose.

The breath for meditation is all important. It is the power tool that will take you into meditation. Take a look at the key points 1-5 below and remember them. They are what will or will not make a difference to your success in meditation.

The breath for meditation should be:

1. Slow

2. Long

3. Even

4. Deep

5. Smooth

These are the key points to remember when learning to meditate. It is well to practise them. As you sit here now, why not practise with me. Make sure you are in a comfortable place, and do not do this whilst you are driving or operating machinery. This exercise is likely to make you go to sleep. It will take away your alertness for a time. We need to be safe and we need to be mindful for meditation. All that having been said, find a comfortable place such as a nice comfy chair, sit in it; and relax. Make sure that you are also in a quiet place where you will not be disturbed for a time. We are not going to go into meditation but will just practice the breathing for meditation. Of course there is a real possibility that you may end up in meditation. This is why we need to be aware of where we are when we do meditation.

Now to begin practising the breath. Take a slow deep breath in, and then slowly breathe out. Do this again and really fill your lungs. Then slowly breathe out. Once again, do the same thing. Slowly breathe in, this time to a count of five. Now let the air out slowly to a count of five. Keep doing this. You will in a short time feel yourself going down into a relaxed state. You will feel yourself feeling calmer and quieter. When you feel yourself become a bit more relaxed and calmer, stop breathing deeply and return to normal breath.

If you did this correctly you will understand that your breathing pattern has an impact on the way that you feel. You will have felt the slight altering of how you feel. You should feel slightly more relaxed, just a little bit calmer. Now practise this many times. Just connect into your breath. Do the exercise at least once a day for a few days so that you become familiar with how it makes you feel when you do it.

A Method for Going into Meditation

Here is a method for going into a deep meditation. There are many methods that will help you to achieve this state, and this is just one of them. This method allows you to just practise focusing on your breathing. It is the breath pattern that will ultimately take you from your alert and awake state to a meditative state. Concentrating on the breath pattern gives the brain a job to do, and thus it will not look for something else to do. It will not wander and start to think about the shopping, work, or the children.

Now you are going to go into a deep meditation. So do the relevant preparations for meditation. Find a safe and comfortable place to sit, a place where you will be undisturbed for the duration of the meditation, such as a comfortable chair. Make yourself comfortable and close your eyes. You are going to relax your body by using the power of your own breath. The breath pattern will change the way you feel, as it will change your brain-wave pattern. As we have learnt previously, this is what takes you down first into relaxation, and then as you go down deeper into relaxation, the breath will take you down into a deep meditation.

1. Close your eyes.

2. Start by taking many slow and deep breaths.

3. Take a deep breath in and really fill your lungs.

4. Slowly breathe out.

5. Start counting slowly to five as you breathe in again.

6. Now hold your breath for a count of three.

7. Now let the breath out slowly to a count of five. Each time you breathe in, really fill your lungs.

8. Consciously feel your body, and allow each part of your body to relax with each and every breath.

9. Work your way up your body, starting with the feet.

10. Breathe in again slowly to a count of five, and as you slowly breathe out, allow your feet to relax.

11. Breathe in again to a count of five and once again fill your lungs.

12. As you breathe out, allow your legs to relax.

13. Breathe in again slowly to a count of five, filling your lungs.

14. Breathe out once again slowly to a count of five, and pull that relaxation up the body to the waist.

15. Breathe in again to a count of five slowly, and breathe out again slowly to a count of five. This time allow the torso to relax.

16. Take another deep breath in to a count of five, and as you breathe out to a count of five, breathe out all tension and allow the body to relax just that little bit further.

17. Feel yourself sinking down, down, down. You are falling downwards, and as you do so you are relaxing completely. Keep breathing slowly to a count of five and keep breathing out to a count of five, and with each inhalation and exhalation you will allow yourself to go down into meditation a little bit deeper. Keep on with this method until a deep meditative state has been achieved.

Once you have achieved the desired state, stay there for a little time. Ten minutes should be ample for the first time. Then slowly bring yourself back from the meditation by focusing on your body.

1. Bring your attention to your feet. Wiggle them and move them.

2. Bring your attention to your legs, and move them also.

3. Bring your attention to your torso, and move your shoulders, your arms, and your hands.

4. Now wake up and open your eyes when you feel ready to do so.

5. Wake up now and come back to the here and the now.

Within meditation we can always bring ourselves back to the here and the now at any stage. We are in control, and even though your subconscious mind has been brought to the fore, your conscious mind will take control should it need to do so. So set that intent before you go into meditation. "I will wake up should there be a need to do so." We are in control at all times.

Spiritual Meditation

The world is awash with different religions and ways of reaching a higher spiritual connection. Each person seeks their own truth in their own way. Some of us will subscribe to one idea or another or one religion or another or no religion at all, depending on what fits best for us. We do not have to follow a religious path to meditate. Meditation can have many purposes, and reaching a higher spiritual truth or spiritual connection is just one of those purposes.

Each of us could live our lives without ever seeking such a connection. Each of us could just go about our everyday tasks and never seek religion at all. Each religion gives us a different take on the world. Each gives us a model for thinking, living, and being within life itself. Each religion promises us a life of enlightenment, contentment, wisdom, and a connection to God if we follow its particular path. There are many people who just wish to follow a path of self-discovery and who wish to find their own way to enlightenment, contentment, wisdom, and God by their own means. These people wish to do so without subscribing to one religion or another. For these people, we have included the first three meditations in this book which are for anyone who wishes to explore the idea of a universal spiritual reality, that Reality that takes you to a higher consciousness, the other reality beyond this one we each share at this moment. Some people strive all of their lives to experience God or to become more of what they perceive God would wish them to be.

If direct communication with God were indeed possible, then all of these people who seek God could commune with and experience that which they seek. I have no idea how these meditations will manifest themselves for you. Each person will have his or her own experiences, as each one of us is different. We are each in different places in our own personal development, and we are all at different junctions on the spiritual path. There are as many places to be as there are people on the planet. It does not matter where you are or where you wish to be. There will be something to be gained if you do these meditations. They are not intended to connect you to your own spiritual self but to connect you to other external spiritual forces. In this way, your own spirit will be nourished. This is food for your soul. Eat well.

May I suggest that you record all of the meditations for your personal use?

It is difficult to do a meditation and to read at the same time. It is possible to put the meditations onto a voice recorder and listen to your own voice sending you into meditation. To gain the maximum from the meditations, remember to leave the correct amount of time between instructions for you to go into meditation. For instance, when it says hold the energy in the solar plexus for five minutes, remember to allow that amount of time on the voice recorder before committing the next instruction to the voice recorder. Give yourself repeated instructions, tell yourself to relax and tell yourself to let go of all tension at the beginning of the recording, and repeat this to yourself many times.

Spirituality is not

A walk in the park,
A walk by the sea,
Sitting by a tree,
Being good,
Being kind,
Anyone there,
Alone in the dark,
A wagging finger,
A sharp tongue,
A straight line,
A clear path,
A lit candle,
A pretty crystal,
A knowledgeable book,
An inspirational speaker.
Instead it's a breeze,
A stillness,
Oneness with spirit,
A journey to the soul.

Lynette Avis

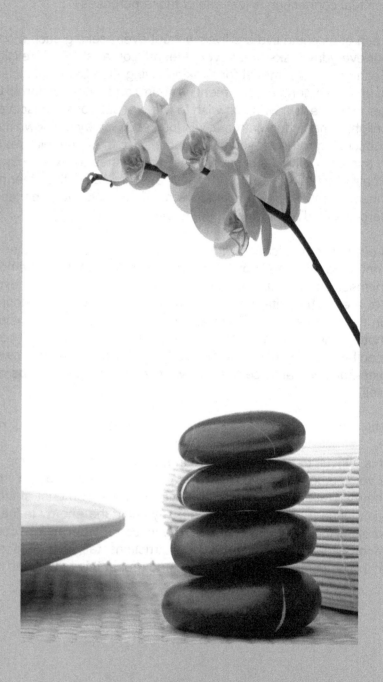

The Recording

Step 1 Start the recording by giving instruction on preparation. Say…

1. I would like you to relax and become comfortable in your chair. Please close your eyes. Just let go of all cares and worries. You do not need them for this time.

2. I would like you to bring your attention to your body. Allow your feet to just sink into the floor. Put your hands on your lap and allow them to relax and sink. Just let go of all tension. I would like you to bring a sense of relaxation up your body. Pull the relaxation up from your feet to your knees. Really let your body sink and let go.

Step 2 Continue the recording with the breathing pattern. Say…

1. Now I would like you to take some really deep breaths in. Really fill your lungs. Now slowly breathe out.

2. We are now going to begin the breathing pattern. So I would like you to slowly breathe in to a count of five. Breath in 1,2,3,4,5. Hold your breath 1,2,3,4,5. Now slowly breath out 1,2,3,4,5.

3. Once again slowly breathe in to a count of five. Breath in 1,2,3,4,5. Hold your breath 1,2,3,4,5. Now slowly breath out 1,2,3,4,5.

4. And again slowly breathe in to a count of five. Breath in 1,2,3,4,5. Hold your breath 1,2,3,4,5. Now slowly breath out 1,2,3,4,5.

5. Again slowly breathe in to a count of five. Breath in 1,2,3,4,5. Now Hold your breath 1,2,3,4,5. slowly breath out 1,2,3,4,5. I would like you to continue your breathing in this way.

6. Now bring your attention back to your body and continue bringing the relaxation up your body. Pull the relaxation up from your knees to your waist.

7. Keep your breath pattern going breathing in deeply 1,2,3,4,5 and now slowly breath out 1,2,3,4,5. Continue bringing relaxation up your body to the tip of your head.

Step 3 Meditation

Place the instructions for the mediation here. Please refer to the instructions of any of the twelve meditations and place those instructions on the recording in this position.Please read the instructions before placing them to get a sense of what needs to be placed on the recording and how.

Step 4 Bring yourself back to the here and the now. Say…

It is now time for you to slowly return. So I would like you to bring your attention and awareness to your body. I would like you to feel your feet. Please wiggle your toes. Now feel your legs and move them. Feel your hands and move your fingers, move your arms. Now move your shoulders and your head. When you feel ready to do so, open your eyes. Wake up now open your eyes and come back to the here and the now. Wake up now open your eyes. You are back in the room and back to the here and the now.

Tips for the Recording

- It is difficult to say how long it will take for any person to fall into meditation. Give at least ten minutes of preparation and relaxation and breathing. It will take some people less time and some people longer to fall into the meditation state. You can adjust your recording to suit your needs. If you are not going off into meditation easily it may be that you need longer at the breathing pattern to take you there or you need to give more instruction to yourself bringing the relaxation up the body. Play with your recording until you get it right for you. Also it is well to note that the more you do the mediations and the meditation preparation process the easier it will become to reach the meditation state. Practise makes perfect. The breath pattern process is the crucial part of the meditation process as it is what will take you into relaxation and on to meditation.

- When it is time to come back to the room give yourself time to come back to the room. It will sometimes take you more time than others to wake up and so include at least five minutes on the recording for the waking up process.

- Make sure that you give the appropriate time between each process when giving the mediation instruction. When a meditation tells you to hold the energy in a place for an amount of minutes you must give that time on the recording. So there has to be the appropriate quite time on the recording corresponding to the mediation instruction.

- When you have gained some experience with mediation and you have learnt to take in deep enough breaths to take you down into meditation you can replace the count of five with a count of three.

- Please refer to the section Set 3 meditations meditation 3 for an example of how to record the mediations.

Set 1: Meditations for Spiritual Connection

Spiritual Meditations Explained

The first three meditations are for everyone and anyone. I would suggest that the very first meditation in this book is for those people who want to communicate with the spiritual reality beyond them. It is for those people who want direct answers and direct speech from the reality beyond this place and this life. Only you can decide if that is for you or not, and only you know why you wish for that communication. So my advice on this very first meditation is to ask yourself why you wish for that communication. Ask yourself, "How will this meditation help me and my life?" This meditation will bring you into direct contact with spirit beings beyond this life and so please think about the possible outcomes of that communication both positive and negative before embarking on this particular meditation.

The first meditation in this set is a good warm-up meditation for platform mediums or for developing mediums. However, as I have said, it is for anyone who wishes to develop a spiritual connection that would allow for direct communication. In fact, it is for anyone who wishes to develop in that way and travel that road. There is much to be gained from travelling the road with spirit, and no one can know what is to be gained on any road unless they, the person in question, are prepared to traverse the path.

The second meditation is a meditation designed to connect you the person to the Universe. It will allow you to feel the Universe and understand your place in it. Who does not want that?

The third meditation is designed to do what we all try to do when we pray or seek religion. It is designed to give you a connection to the ultimate power of the Universe. It is designed to connect you to that which some call "God", some "the God force", and some "the ultimate power of all that there is". How you choose to think of that force or power is your choice. This third meditation is designed to take you to that power. Happiness is bliss. Enjoy the experience.

Meditation 1: Direct Communication with Spirit Energy

1. Go into relaxation.

2. Bring energy into the body from the crown of the head.

3. Take the energy down to the solar plexus.

4. Hold the energy in the solar plexus for ten minutes.

5. Bring energy up to the throat and then hold at the throat for ten minutes.

6. Next bring the energy down to the solar plexus once again and hold here for just five minutes.

7. Take the energy back up to the crown for two minutes.

8. Now send the energy out of the crown to the Universe to connect for direct communication with spirit energy.

This is the process that is used to connect to spirit. This will take you down through the layers of consciousness for direct communication with spirit beings beyond your own spirit.

Please refer to the section of Chapter 3 entitled "The Seven Major Chakra Points" for information on chakras and their positions in the body.

Meditation 2: Universal Connection to the Collective Consciousness

1. Bring in energy to the body through the crown of the head.

2. Now slowly take it through the chakra energy points (the crown, third eye, throat, heart, solar plexus, sacral, and base).

3. Leave the energy in each point for about three minutes.

4. Go through the all of the chakra points. Activation of the whole system is important here.

5. Once the whole system has been activated, bring the energy back up to the solar plexus and allow the energy to sit there for five minutes. This will fill the solar plexus and fully activate this point.

6. Now slowly send out the energy in a slow and steady flow to the Universe.

7. Keep the flow slow and measured.

8. Imagine now there is a continuous and steady flow of energy between yourself and the Universe.

9. Energy comes in from the top of your head and out through your solar plexus. The stream is continuous and endless.

10. Now feel connected to the collective consciousness.

Meditation 3: Connection to the God Force

1. Bring energy in through the top of the head.

2. Bring energy down to the solar plexus slowly in steps and stages.

3. Now allow the energy to sit at this point for three to five minutes.

4. Now imagine the energy is flowing faster and faster out to the Universe. It moves further and further away from you to the extremes of the Universe, and as it does so it connects to all that there is.

5. You are now connected to the God force.

"True silence is the rest of the mind, and is to the spirit what sleep is to the body, nourishment and refreshment."

William Penn

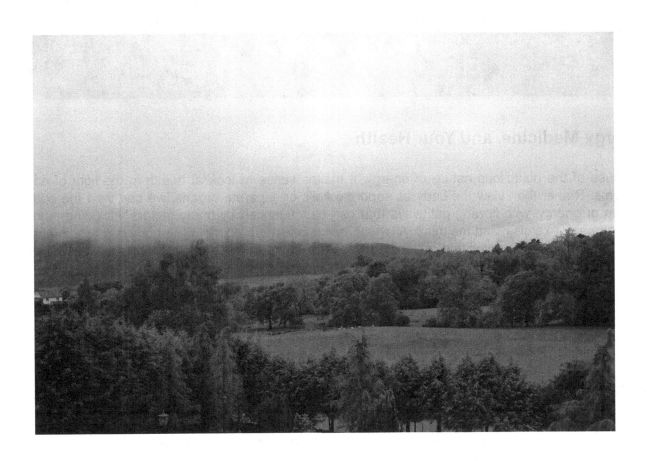

Energy Medicine, and Your Health

Because of the ubiquitous nature of energy, it makes sense to look at health in the light of energy systems. Rather than view the body as separate cells or separate organs, we can view the body as a form of energy, with flowing pathways that can be influenced by many factors, including nutrition, environment, exercise, and the mind. All these things affect our energy. The body is a fully integrated whole, each system affecting and influencing all the others in a delicate balance that, if maintained, leads to full health, vitality, and a fulfilling living experience. We will have the energy to meet the challenges of life, to put our energy into what we feel is important to us, to work, to rest, and to play.

Advances in modern western science have been phenomenal. Endless money has been ploughed into research into so many areas of medicine. And yet we have not found cures for cancer or AIDS, and we are stunningly naive about the workings of the body, the immune system, and our health in general. Western medicine initially progressed through the study of the dead body, and this has developed into research that uses cell culture in an attempt to reproduce the human living environment. It is a start, but we have to acknowledge that the human body is incredibly complex. Though we may find answers by trying to break it down and simplify the conditions, the fact is that the human body works as a whole, not as individual cells, organs, or parts. By studying it in its entirety, we may begin to unravel its infinite complexity. Eastern health practices, such as Ayurvedic medicine or traditional Chinese medicine (TCM) took the body as a whole—and not as an isolated whole either. The environment, the people, and the activities, as well as the diet and the mental health of the person, were all considered. Even the time of the year and astrological readings were taken into account. It was understood that the body was part of a greater whole from which we are inseparable.

Energy is part of that system—part of the problem and the cure—for we are made of matter, and matter is energy. We even talk in English of being "low in energy", feeling "energised", "flat", "bubbly" or "excited", to name a few expressions that show that we think of ourselves in this way. We think of ourselves as having energy as a living, integral part of the system that is us. So many of these traditional medicines talked of energy as the building block or foundation of everything, spawning the disciplines of acupuncture, acupressure, Reiki, meridians and chi manipulation, meditation itself, and so on. Ayurvedic doctors believed the body was made from consciousness (energy), and therefore they practised a medicine of consciousness, whereby the healing came from the mind. The foundation of the Universe is one of balance, and the energy of the body, as of all nature, needs to sustain equilibrium. Ill health is a manifestation of imbalance, brought about by stresses of various kinds. Redressing these imbalances brings about natural healing.

It is as if there is an intelligence built within the system that harnesses the strength and vitality that is abundant in nature herself. Interfere with this balance through poor sleep and diet, sustained stress without appropriate relaxation, or negative belief and value structures, and ill health, as well as poor recovery or no recovery at all, will inevitably result.

The influence of the mind on the body through the brain is well documented. Thoughts release neuropeptides and neurotransmitters from the brain throughout the body, affecting it in many ways. Sustained signals of stress, brought about by the fight or flight response, have adverse effects on almost every cell of the body, while signals of relaxation, created through meditation or walking in a wood in nature, have positive effects on almost all the cells in the body. The idea of the "mind- body", which suggests that a seamless connection exists between the mind and the body, may help to explain the extraordinary recoveries cited by Deepak Chopra in many of his books, as well as those in *The Healing Codes* by Alexander Loyd and Ben Johnson.

It is through the acceptance of these ideas by such Western-trained physicians that the barriers of Western medicine are beginning to open up and consider many of these medical practises. Seen from the view of "living energy", it makes perfect sense that medicine should work with energy, the life force, and consider its balance and well-being as an integral part of patient care.

Remember, illness is part of the quantum soup as well. It is a product of that source. To view it as the "enemy" is ultimately to go about it in a negative way. We must be kind. We must be calm and relaxed and redress balance. Once the energy system is in balance, the source of the manifestation of illness disappears, and the illness and its symptoms vanish. Perhaps part of the success of this way of healing is based upon the discipline of the mind that heals. A poorly disciplined mind will have less success than a disciplined mind. An ill-disciplined mind has scattered energy, while a disciplined mind has focussed energy, energy that can bring the energy of the body back into equilibrium.

What is the mind? We think of the mind as the brain, the cells, and the chemicals within them that transmit the electrical impulses that result in the subconscious functioning of the body (breathing, heartbeat, balance, digestion, the immune system, homeostasis, etc.), movement, thought, and creation. Trace a movement or a thought back to its source, and what do you find? Chemicals? Electricity? Or are these the first steps in a series of steps that started with something less material? In short, where does thought come from? The chemicals and the electricity are used to transmit the thought, but the thought itself? What if the thought itself comes from this quantum soup? What if it is the source—that which starts the whole process? A thought coming from this source simply manifests itself physically in the brain and ultimately in the body. It is as if the brain can be a receiver for such things, if it is allowed to be, if it is calm enough, at peace and in tranquillity. But there are in fact two sources.

One is this deep source, the energy, the quantum soup that possesses the wisdom of the Universe across time. In TCM the Chinese refer to this as "chi", while in Ayurvedic medicine, a Hindu tradition, it is called "prana". It enlivens the body and keeps it strong and healthy. In TCM methods, such as herbal remedies, acupuncture, massage, chi kung, and t'ai chi, are used to restore harmony to the body so that the chi energy can flow naturally and freely and so maintain health at a physical, mental, and spiritual level. In Ayurvedic medicine, energy balance is also an essential part of maintaining health in similar ways to TCM. The American Indians refer to it as "medicine", the power of the Universe that keeps the human body healthy and in balance. It is part of a universal whole, and if we allow ourselves, we can be healed by this universal power, kept healthy by it, and made whole by its grace. In some yoga forms, pranayama is the practice in which the control of prana is initially achieved from the discipline of one's breathing. According to yogic philosophy, the breath or air is merely a gateway to the world of prana and its manifestation in the body. In yoga, pranayama techniques are used to control the movement of these vital energies within the body, which is said to lead to an increase in vitality in the practitioner. In short, these different practices gain access to this quantum soup to aid healing. They give it different names, but it is the same thing, rejuvenating the body and bringing it back into balance, so that the universal energy can flow unhindered, sustaining health in mind, body, and spirit.

The second source is the energy that is put into our minds by learning. The thoughts and ideas of parents, siblings, peers, and teachers enter our minds from a very early age. These are the values, beliefs, and principles that guide and direct us in our life's journey. But they are not ours. They are put there, and we believe them to be ours. These thoughts steer our lives and make us see the world in a particular way. They make us see life, health, disease, and ageing from a certain standpoint. Thoughts from generations past live on within us as they are passed from parent to child.

In the case of disease, perhaps we find ourselves ill and view it in a negative way, making the symptoms worse. In the normal flow of events, the body is exposed to a bacteria or a virus, and the immune system recognises it as something harmful and leaps into action to remove it from the body. This is literally happening all the time. Yet when illness takes hold, especially a severe disease like cancer, we become fearful and even depressed, flooding the body with negative thoughts that have an overall detrimental effect on the entire body. The energy of fear rather than the energy of healing enters all the cells of the body, and it makes it harder for the body to heal. There are many documented cases of dramatic recoveries from terminal diseases, but they are so infrequent and so beyond the explanations of conventional medicine that they are dismissed.

We can choose the source of the energy that powers our mind and our body. Either we choose the universal source with all its wisdom and infinite knowledge, or we choose the learned source with its incumbent prejudices and limited understanding. Meditation takes us to the universal source, allowing us to connect to the healing power of the Universe. Reiki practitioners use this power to heal people, just as acupuncture releases blockages of this power to allow the body to regain balance and harmony.

Taking our power from the learned source leaves us with our prejudiced thoughts, moving our attention away from the universal energy and keeping our focus on our limited understanding of the way of things. Though it is all energy, it is the quality of that energy that is the key. The negative energy from thoughts of worry, anxiety, and stress has a negative effect on our health. We know, for example, that prolonged stress reduces the effectiveness of the immune system. Positive thoughts of relaxation, calm, and compassion have a positive effect on our health. We know that mindfulness meditation connects us to a calm and tranquillity that leads to better and more congruent brain function, as well as to a more relaxed and supple body and improved immune response.

Western medicine's body of knowledge has been built upon clinical trials that attempt to truly define the effects of treatments upon the patient. Until recently, this has not been the manner of conducting trials in TCM and Ayurvedic medicine. However, trials exposed to the rigors of controls, double blinds, randomisation, placebos and nocebos are increasing in Ayurvedic and particularly in TCM circles. They can only help to establish their credibility in the eyes of Western medicine. Practitioners are finding ways to satisfy Western medicine's scientific rigour and at the same time remain true to the founding principles and ideas of their art. [1]

But we are all different. Each one of us is on a different journey and at a different point along that journey. These subtle differences make a huge difference in relation to diagnosis and curative methods. Every stage of our lives affects us and affects the energy of our being, and so this must affect the body as well as the mind. Ill health is simply an imbalance in that energy. The body and mind are out of kilter, and that imbalance manifests in poor health.

The effects of meditation have been well documented by Western medicine. Meditation is shown to have great positive effects in combating stress and therefore the effects of stress—not just stress in daily living, but also the stress that comes with ill health. It is well documented that stressful living

---

[1] Mathur, A., and V. Sankar. "Standards of Reporting Ayurvedic Clinical Trials. Is There a Need?" Journal of Ayurveda and Integrative Medicine, Vol 1, Issue 1, pages 52- 55. Reprinted by permission of Medknow Publications

can lead to suppressed immune response and therefore increase our likelihood of becoming ill, while recovery from serious illnesses such as HIV and cancer can be impaired when the patient is stressed or depressed as a result of their condition. Mindfulness-based stress reduction (MBSR) uses meditation as part of its technique to reduce stress. Studies using magnetic resonance images have shown that meditation can promote growth in structures in the brain involved in learning, memory, self-awareness, compassion and introspection, correlating to an improvement in these qualities, while meditation also appears to reduce the size of areas of the brain associated with anxiety and stress, with a corresponding reduction in these behaviours.[2] Improved recovery after treatment for HIV and breast cancer has also been found to be significant when patients undergo MBSR.[3]

The meditations in this chapter, along with the others in this book, will help to redress the imbalances, if any. This does not mean that they are a cure for all ills, and we would recommend consulting a doctor or other health professional if you suspect any signs of ill health. What we are saying is that the energy of the Universe is the same as the energy in our bodies. Nature's way is to maintain balance. This energy interacts with itself all the time, and we are a part of that interaction, so we must consider the whole of our lives and the whole of our experience when we look at our "selves" as an energy form. Health is a manifestation of that balance, while imbalance will ultimately result in ill health of some kind. Western medicine often seeks to mask the source of ill health by treating the symptoms, rather than looking at the source itself, the quantum soup, and finding ways to harness it and promote good health and so deal with the symptoms too. Perhaps we need to look at our whole life when we look at health in this way. Our whole life affects our energy, and so masking the problem only leads to greater imbalance. Ill health is telling us there is something wrong, that we need to make a change. The source will interact with us, help us, guide us, and help heal us as we seek to help and heal ourselves.

[2] Britta K. Hölzel, James Carmody, Mark Vangel, Christina Congleton, Sita M. Yerramsetti, Tim Gard, and Sara W. Lazar. "Mindfulness practice leads to increases in regional brain gray matter density." Psychiatry Research: Neuroimaging, 2011; 191 (1): 36).
[3] Yaowarat Matchim, Jane M. Armer, Bob R. Stewart. December 2011. "Effects of Mindfulness-Based Stress Reduction (MBSR) on Health among Breast Cancer Survivors," Western Journal of Nursing Research, Vol 33, Issue 8, pages 996- 1016.

The Subtle Energy System

The word "chakra" is the Sanskrit word for "wheel" or "circle" and also means "wheel of light". The chakra positions come from the Hindu spiritual practice, and are locations of energy within the body. The chakra points are also said to be spinning wheels of energy that spin in opposite directions from each other, going up the body from the base chakra point, which is located at the base of the spine. They are in fact centres of energy within the body located at the main branching of the nervous system. They run in a line along the body from the base of the spine to the top of the head. There are many differing authorities on chakra knowledge. However, mostly they all agree that the chakras are converging lines of energies within the body.

We do not think of the body in this way in the West. We think of the body as a series of organs, blood, flesh, and bones. We do not think of the body in terms of energy that travels around the body and spins.

The chakras are part of what is known as the subtle energy body. It is the energy circulatory system of the person or the system by which the universal energy travels around the physical body. It is a bit like our blood circulatory system. Some spiritual disciplines also say that we have three bodies—our physical body, our spiritual body, and our subtle energy body.

The energy travels to the various organs by way of this energy circulatory system, which in the Hindu belief system is called "nadis", thus regulating the various organs as they are fed by the energy circulating around the system. This is very similar to blood circulation that also feeds the body by taking various necessities around the body. There are many people in the West who are sceptical of the existence of this energy system. It is hard to prove that it exists at all within the body.

To feel the subtle energy/universal energy travelling within the body is not a difficult thing to achieve. The practice of chi kung is a good way of feeling the energy travelling around the body. The exercises within chi kung are very simple and will very quickly send the energy around the body, and it can be felt very easily. If there is a blockage, it will be very quickly felt by the person within the execution of the simple exercises within chi kung. People in China who practice chi kung regularly are said to live very long and healthy lives. We can also feel this energy moving around the body if we have a Reiki treatment or various other holistic energy treatments. Within a Reiki treatment, the energy will be felt as hot or cold, as dull energy or sometimes as pain either within the body or travelling through the body. It is a very definite feeling and is not just in the person's head. It is felt as physical feeling.

For our purposes within this book, it does not matter if the chakras spin or not. What matters is that you understand their location. For that is what a chakra occupies—a location on and within the body. Just as your heart and lungs and liver occupy a position and a place within the body, so too do the chakras. I realize I am giving a very simple explanation of the chakras in this book. The chakras are a large subject in themselves, and there are a great number of books that deal with them in depth from all angles and aspects and belief systems. Within this book you do not have to subscribe to any way of thinking on the subject of chakras or gain any great knowledge about them. To do the meditations correctly, you will need to know where the specific points are. So it will be well to learn the chakra positions. It matters within the meditations where the energy is taken to within the body, what duration it is held for, and at what point this is done in the various meditations. That is part of what will bring the desired results within the meditations. If you take the energy to the wrong places for the wrong duration, you will not achieve what you are seeking within each meditation.

We can influence the energy with the power of our minds alone. We do not have to do anything complicated at all. Just understand that the energy will move when you tell it to do so with your mind.

Just imagining the energy travelling along the various chakras will make it do so. The energy travels around your body all of the time without any thought from you at all, and it will do so also with just the power of your will. You can grow the energy within the various chakra points, and you can send the energy out from various chakra points that you choose. The energy will flow when you make it do so and how you make it do so.

The more you practise taking the energy up and down the chakra points, the more connection to the chakras and the energy you will have on a conscious level. You will feel the energy more and more. We are all different individuals, and we all differ in all things. Some will find this easy to do and will take to it like a duck to water, while others will struggle with connecting into the feeling of the energy. It is like all things: the more we practise, the better we will get at it. It is not a huge learning curve to connect to the energy.

Just practise it a little, and you will eventually understand that you are moving the energy. Remember the word "subtle" when you are manipulating the energy. The energy is subtle, and therefore it will take some concentration on the energy to enable yourself to eventually feel the energy. It is easy to feel a hammer falling on your toe. It is not so easy to feel a feather.

I give some basic information on the seven main chakra points just to help you in some basic understanding of them, as I know there will be many of you reading this book that have no knowledge of the chakras at all.

When one knows that the Great Void is full of ch'i, one realises that there is no such thing as nothingness.

—Chang Tsai

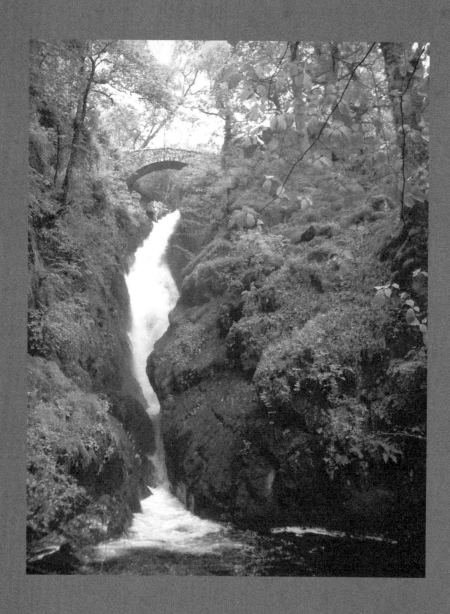

The Seven Major Chakra Points

The seven major chakra points are shown below.

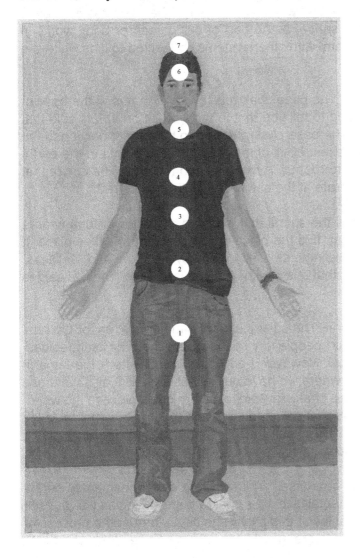

7. The crown
6. The third eye
5. The throat
4. The heart
3. The solar plexus
2. The sacral
1. The base

The seven major chakra points run from the base of the spine to the top of the head.

If I asked you where your heart is, would you know the answer? I am sure most of us have felt our own hearts. We all know where our heart is, and so we know where the heart chakra is. It is the heart itself. We know the heart exists, we know it pumps blood, and we know it is powered somehow as it keeps pumping. Something is fuelling its movement. It is a centre of energy. The energy of the heart just keeps on going. Thank goodness for that! As long as it keeps on going, we know we are alive and well.

Now if I asked you where your throat is, would you know where the answer? Of course you do. It is inside your neck, and it holds your voice box that allows you to make lots of sounds. The sound that comes out of that throat of yours is energy. So there we have our centre of energy at the throat chakra position. Is there a spinning wheel of energy there? I do not know any more than you. I know that it is a point of energy, and that is what matters for our purposes within this book. Similarly, each of the other chakra points has energy. At each position something or other happens within you energetically. At your crown you have thoughts at the third eye and you see pictures. Now I would like you to imagine a giraffe. Where did you see the picture of the giraffe? At your third eye or brow position, I bet. So there we have it; there is energy activity there. I could go on, but I am sure you take my point.

Each of the chakras has a function on a physical and a psychological level, and they are also said to be interconnected with our organs and the endocrine system which is the system that secretes hormones within the body. To me this makes a great deal of sense, as no part of our person or body works in total isolation. Our body is a complete physical system, with other systems connected to it as well—the spiritual and the energetic.

The chakras go up the body from the base chakra. The base chakra is the point that is at the base of your body, and to understand its true location I need to tell you that in fact you sit on it. It is said that all chakras go up the body from the base chakra. The base chakra is said to be our connection to the earth. It is situated at the base of the spine. It is closest of all of the major chakra points to the earth, and so that makes sense. This chakra is also said to root us in the here and the now. The colour that this chakra is given is red. This chakra is said to vibrate at the same rate as the colour red.

Moving up from the base chakra, the next chakra is the sacral. It is situated at the lower tummy area just above the groin. This chakra is our creative seat. It is the place where procreation takes place. It is the place of the life force. It is said to determine feelings, sexuality, intimacy, passion, and liveliness. This chakra is all about sexual harmony. The colour that this chakra is given is orange, and it is said to vibrate at the same rate as the colour orange.

The solar plexus is the next chakra up from the sacral. The solar plexus is situated just under the bust area or in the equivalent placement on a man. Some people say this is where the soul itself resides. Who knows? Perhaps or perhaps not. I do not know. However, I do know this: is where I feel that it resides when in I am in meditation. This is certainly where we have our gut feelings. We all have those from time to time, and this is where we feel them. This chakra is said to govern one's place in the world, one's self-esteem, and one's control of oneself, personal power, desire, and touch. On a mental level, this chakra is said to stimulate intellectual faculties. The colour that this chakra is given is yellow, and it is said to vibrate at the same rate as the colour yellow.

The heart is the next chakra. This is situated at the heart itself. This is where our connection to others resides, our feelings of love and connection. On a mental level, this chakra helps us to validate our self and also our relationships with others. On a spiritual level, this chakra helps us to trust the process of life and evolution. The colour that this chakra is given is green, and it is said to vibrate at the same rate as the colour green.

The next chakra is the throat. This is the seat of communication, and I can definitely attest to that. Lots of sound comes from this area on my body—some will say too much, but let's not go there! This chakra is said to be where we identify our own needs and verbalise them to others. It is said that having this chakra in good working order on a spiritual level can result in clairaudience for mediums. Clairaudience is the ability to hear spirits that have passed to the other side of life, or in other words, people who are now dead to this world and living in the next world. Energising this chakra and doing the meditation on spirit communication will be a valuable development tool for any developing medium. The colour that this chakra is given is blue, and it is said to vibrate at the same rate as the colour blue.

The brow or third eye is the next chakra up from the throat. This is the place where we see pictures in our mind. This chakra facilitates insight and visualization. On a mental level, this is where the ability to perceive beyond the five senses lies and our ability to link with intuition. This is the place of true power and true knowledge. On a physical level, this is said to govern the pituitary gland, which is the gland at the back of the head that governs the production of hormones from all other glands. The colour that this chakra is given is indigo, and it is said to vibrate at the same rate as the colour indigo.

The crown chakra is the final chakra. It is the chakra that is associated with wisdom and spiritual connection. It is the chakra nearest to the heavens, and it is through this chakra that we receive higher wisdom and knowledge. The colour that this chakra is given is violet, and it is said to vibrate at the same rate as the colour violet.

I think that when we talk about the energy system, we have to be aware of the fact that there are many theories. There is no one hard and fast right or wrong. Many cultures have tried to explain what they felt to be true with regard to how the energy enters and flows through our bodies. The energy system is like all things that man has taken his curious mind to. It is there to be investigated and understood. Eventually the complete truth of how it works and what it is will be understood by mankind. It merely takes time and a curious mind.

The Aura

In my educational journey on spirituality and energy, I have been taught many things. I have been taught by some that the aura is an electromagnetic phenomenon and by others that the aura holds the spark of life itself—that it is our very soul. I think we can all split hairs and argue about this until the cows come home, but what proof can we give about the aura being the very soul of a person that would completely satisfy everyone? I had a student who came to me two years ago and said that he wanted me to teach him about the aura amongst other things. This student wanted me to prove to him that the aura exists. The fact is that it is easy to prove that the aura exists. You can feel your own aura. That is proof enough for most people. When people feel the subtle energy that emanates from their own bodies with their own hands, they are on the road to understanding.

The Subtle Energy

The subtle energy that exudes from our bodies is called the aura. It is believed to be an electromagnetic energy, so we can say it is both electric and magnetic and that in that capacity it can indeed be measured by scientists with the right equipment. So what more proof of the aura do any of us need? The aura is there, and we can feel it; we can measure it, and some people can also see it. Not all people can see the aura. In fact, I have been one of those people who struggle with seeing the aura. However, I know I feel the quality of other people's auras, and so I trust this ability to feel that quality. Like all of us, I can feel the colours that exist within a person's aura, but we do not all understand consciously that we are doing this. We all do this subconsciously. I have done numerous exercises with my teachers in the past, who have shown me that I can feel the difference in quality from one person to another and that it is a reality and not in my head. The exercises are simple to do, they are very revealing, and to some students they are quite eye opening. They were so to me, and they are so to many of the people I have taught. I have given some of these exercises here for you to try.

Feeling Your Own Aura

1. Roll your sleeve up and expose your arm.

2. First I want you to feel for the heat that comes out of your body naturally. So put the palm of your other hand just about two or three inches away from the exposed skin of the exposed arm and feel for your natural body heat. Register how that feels and take your hand away.

3. Now once again bring your hand towards your arm. This time start much higher above the arm—about eighteen inches away from the arm. Now slowly lower the hand towards the exposed arm. As you do so, register what you are feeling or sensing in the palm of your hand.

You may have to do this several times very slowly before you feel anything at all. You will feel a very subtle difference in the area surrounding your arm as you lower your palm to your arm. The difference felt is often said to be a spongy resistance, and that is what you are looking for. It will be very subtle, but once have felt it, you will always feel it.

Feeling the Aura of Another Person

1. Stand with the person whose aura you are reading in front of you.

2. Now place your palms in front of you and just about one to two feet from the person.

3. Move your palms towards the person until you feel the resistance of the aura. Now feel the aura all around the person.

See the Aura by Relaxing your Eyes

Stand your person in front of a wall that is plain and blank. A white wall would be ideal. Now stand about five or six feet away from your person. Relax your eyes by taking them out of focus. Now look at the person with your eyes out of focus and look just to the right or left of the person or above the person a little way to see the aura. The aura may extend about two feet. You may experience seeing the aura as just grey, or you even see the aura as colour. Now look around the person's aura and note the colours at different points of the aura. The colours will probably be close to the person's body. Look at a distance between two and eight inches from the body. Ask the person to think of a time they were happy and take note of the change in the aura. Ask them to think of a time they were sad. Once again take note of the change in the aura. Now say something to make them laugh. Take note of any colour changes in the aura.

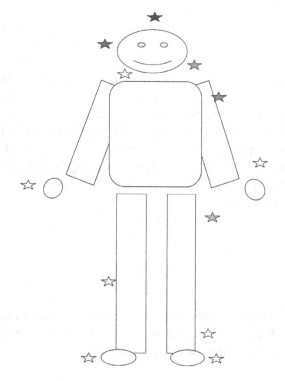

Draw a simple image of a person on your paper. Look around the edges of the person, a few inches or so to see the aura.

Look around the edges of the person for the colours of the aura. By relaxing your eyes, you may see the aura as moving energy like the fuel being burned at the back of an aeroplane, or you may see the colours of the aura.

Sensing or Seeing the Colour of the Aura.

You will need some paper and some coloured pencils and a willing friend to help you. Draw a simple figure of a person on your paper. Now place your friend against a plain background, either a light colour or a dark colour. Now take your eyes out of focus and look around the person's body and see if you can detect any energy emanating from them. Look at the area just outside of the physical body to the side of your person about one or two inches away from the person. Look around the body and mark on your drawing where you see colour with your pencils. If like me you are not good at seeing the colour within the energy, try to see what colours you feel are there. Do not confer with anyone who is doing the exercise with you.

This exercise works best when you have many people doing it at once, as you can confer when you have finished the exercise. Do not confer whilst doing the exercise. At the end of the exercise compare your results and see where you have seen or felt the colours to be and what colours were seen or felt where. You may be surprised to see that most people, if not all of you, will have very similar colours results.

Even if we do not know we are reading the colours that the person is giving out within the aura, we are actually doing so all of the time. We all see, sense, and feel the auras of other living beings. We can detect a great deal of information about the person or other living being by the condition of the aura. We are all giving out information about ourselves to others all of the time through our auras and the condition of our energy system. If the energy system is in poor health, this will show in the condition of the aura first and then will eventually show in the condition of the physical body. Our bodies are giving us information all of the time about what is well and what is not so well with us on all levels of our being. When we train ourselves to read auras by feel or vision, we can gain information that can be used in helping people who are ill. However, once a person trains themselves to do so consciously, there is much more information to be read in the aura other than just the physical health of the individual. We all read each other's auras subconsciously all of the time. We feel each other as well as seeing each other.

Physical Health

Last night I went to bed very late and had little sleep. I stayed up to watch a period drama on TV. I had to get up very early, as my builder wanted to bring the carpenter around to have a look at the work that I need to be done to my house. What has that got to do with health? Well, I am basically tired and a bit fuzzy-headed. My body is not working efficiently, and I really feel like going back to bed for a few hours' sleep. The time is now 11.30 a.m.—not even midday, and I am ready for bed.

There is no one to blame for this poor state of affairs but myself and the TV company for putting the drama on so late. Of course I could have recorded the drama, but our recorder is not connected to the TV as my husband removed it. Don't ask. I know, I know. Let's not go there. So here I am writing about health, and I feel terrible myself. My brain won't work and my body wants a rest. We all need adequate rest to stay healthy. We need to go to bed and get in our full six to eight hours of sleep as is recommended by doctors. I am not sure how many hours I had, but it was not that many. Now it is okay to do what I did one or twice every now and again, but we all know that if we deprive ourselves of our beauty sleep, we will not be in a very beautiful state in the long run.

According to the NHS health advice web site, there are lots of reasons, other than not going to bed at an appropriate time, for persistent tiredness. There could be underlying health issues such as anaemia or an underactive thyroid gland that need to be addressed. So it is wise and appropriate to seek the advice of one's GP to make sure this is not the case.

Tiredness is a real health issue at the moment in Britain. My builder, the carpenter, and I were talking today about stress and how each of us had at some point in our lives suffered with it. Stress and tiredness can be linked together. The NHS Web site says, "At any given time, one in five people feels unusually tired, and one in ten have prolonged fatigue, according to the Royal College of Psychiatrists. Women tend to feel tired more than men." The web site further says, "It's unusual to find anything physically wrong. Most of the time, fatigue is linked with mood and the accumulation of lots of little stresses in life."

I know from experience that being over-stressed and deprived of sleep can lead to ill health in the long run. I went down that road many years ago and paid for it with my health. I had ME for many years, and looking back now, I would say it was due to doing too much work, worrying too much, and a lack of sleep for many years. I did not consider the effects that over-work and working at times when I should have been asleep would have on my body and my life. I did not consider that my body, emotions, and mind are just not made for that kind of abuse. So many of us now are chasing the economic rainbow. We chase that elusive pot of gold that will set us right for the good life or old age. We juggle work, friends, family, study, two jobs, the house, home life, hobbies (if we have time for them), and whatever else we can pack in. No wonder we are all stressed-out wrecks.

The NHS Web site says that at least a third of us are sleep-deprived due to money or job concerns and that psychological tiredness is far more common than tiredness that's caused by a physical problem. They say that anxiety can cause insomnia and in turn lead to persistent fatigue. Well, the conversation that I had today with my builder and carpenter can support that theory. I can contest to that theory. When I was younger, I worried about everything. I did so for years. I think that I just got into a habit of worry, and I never ever stood still long enough to take note of what I was doing to myself.

I suppose I can trace some of my worrying back to my teens, when my father became bankrupt. I think that was the start of it for me. I had to strive to do well and to make a life for myself. I worked hard, and when there was overtime at work, I usually took the opportunity to earn the extra money required to move my life forward. Life and life's choices are far from easy.

Obesity is another hot health issue in Britain today, as it is in much of the Western world. When I was a child, the issue of childhood obesity was not debated. In fact, food and weight were debated at the other extreme. How to make sure that all children obtained the correct nourishment so that they were not malnourished or underfed was the uppermost concern. My mother, who was born in 1927, would tell me about when she was a young girl and the lack of food that she had to endure during her childhood. My mother was brought up by her grandmother and grandfather during the war years. They were not rich people, just ordinary folk. My grandfather's job was to cut the hedgerows in his village and surrounding areas. In those days it was done by hand. It was very physical work, and I am sure it was back-breaking stuff.

They were frugal people, but without enough money frugality will do no good. My mother would tell my sisters and me when we were children how she would more often than not come home to a supper of bread and cheese. That was on the good nights. On the bad ones it was an empty stomach and hunger to take to bed with her. My mother told us how she had holes in her shoes and would have to put cardboard in them to keep out the water and dirt. My mother had a hard life, but probably no harder and in fact better than some. My mother-in-law, who was of the same age give or take one or two years, had a harder and more deprived childhood. My mother-in-law was very malnourished, and that had a long-term impact on her health and body.

Even today there is a relationship between wealth, food, and health. People in the West have become richer over the past few decades. We are now told by the medics that we have an obesity problem. Sometimes obesity has a relationship to eating incorrectly and not just to eating too much. Whichever way one looks at the problem, it is a problem of calories in relation to expenditure of energy. Many people who are the least well off will eat foods that provide calories rather than good nutrition, as some foods are out of their financial reach.

Past generations had jobs that required them to be physical, as my great grandfather did. Many more people work in jobs today that require them to be sedentary for long periods of time. That too has its impact on health. We walk less than we did in the past, and we drive and ride in vehicles in preference to using our legs.

I am a child of the fifties, and by the time I was born life had become a little better. We always had food, and I did not go hungry as a child. I am not saying that it was turkey every day or smoked salmon and wine in our house—not at all. However, we had good food and a meal each day, together with breakfast and tea. The food we had was wholesome and simple, the sort of English cooking that has almost disappeared—toad in the hole, bubble and squeak, meat pies and meat puddings, chops, and mince. For desert there was apple crumbles and cornflake tarts, rice puddings, jam tarts, and spotted dick and custard.

On my father's side, there was rice and peas and chicken on Sundays, salt cod fish and onions, yams and sweet potatoes, and green bananas and plantains to eat. I was never fond of sweet potatoes and still am not. My father would always impart his wisdom on nutrition. He would talk about his mother and all she had taught him on the subject of cooking back home in Jamaica. My father was all for pulses, and to this day I love them. I could eat them until they came out of my ears. He would make us wholesome soups on Saturdays. He would throw into the pot everything that was good for you. He would put in lentils, pulses, vegetables of every kind, including lots of dark green vegetables for iron. He would start with, say, neck of lamb or a cut of meat that was cheap, and then he would add the other ingredients in steps and stages and leave all to simmer and cook. It has been a trend that many people in Britain today just do not know how to cook the most basic of dishes. They don't cook or they can't cook. Times and expectations have changed on many things. Cooking and food habits have been no exception to the changes in daily life for many.

There have been changes that are for the better in society, but I would argue that not being able to cook is to leave oneself lacking and short of a basic and vital life skill. I think this loss of skill by so many people is due to the fact that many women went to work from the sixties onwards. Juggling the demands of home, family and a working life has taken its toll on women and society and health and nutrition in general. When I brought up my own son in the eighties, food seemed to change. We become dependent on supermarkets for all of our produce. More and more, we bought packet foods and went for convenience over nutrition. I am not sure how wise this was, but in the light of current thinking about the quality of ingredients that went into processed foods at that time (the eighties and nineties), it was probably not so wise.

Anyone who has grown their own vegetables will know that the taste of home-grown vegetables cannot be beaten. In the early eighties my partner at that time grew all of our vegetables, and I still think of that time. The taste of those vegetables was flavourful and sweet. Shop-bought vegetables are grown with resistance to pests and disease and with speed and quantity in mind. Famers have to produce for the planet's population and for profit. We do lose a bit of nutritional value and taste in the requirement of the other considerations. Swings and roundabouts, I suppose. However, we can all take control over what goes into our own mouths. We choose what we purchase and how we spend our time. Not everyone can grow their own vegetables. It is not possible or practical for many people. Many people lead such busy lives or live in the city these days. It is not an option to cook everything fresh or to grow one's own food. This is a shame, because so much good nutrition is lost by not doing so.

We are in control of whether we eat vegetables or not. We are urged by the medical profession all of the time to eat more vegetables and to eat less fat and salt. It seems that this message is not getting through, as so many people are ill because of poor diet and poor food choices. The UK's obesity statistics are enumerated by the NHS as follows.

- In 2008, the latest year with available figures, nearly a quarter of adults (over sixteen years of age) in England were obese (had a BMI over thirty). Just under a third of women (thirty-two per cent) were overweight (a BMI of 25-30), and forty-two per cent of men were overweight.

- Amongst children between two and fifteen years of age, one in six boys and one in seven girls in England were obese in 2008. The number of overweight children was also around one in seven.

- The number of overweight and obese people is likely to increase. The Foresight Report, a scientific report used to guide government policy, has predicted that by 2025 nearly half of men and over a third of women will be obese.

In my parents' generation before the war, money and the affordability of food kept food scarce. That generation was much more physically active than my generation or my son's generation. We all rely on machines to do heavy labour or labour in general. We ride in vehicles rather than walk. Perhaps we should all be walking more and making the effort to do more generally by way of making our bodies move and being much more active. This is a message that has been pounded to death by the medical profession, with good cause. It's clear we are not all getting their message. The statistics above are horrible. Change is built into living and life. It is built into our physical bodies. We live, we grow old, and we die. That is fact. We do not have to hasten the fact. We can take care of ourselves in the middle bit of that truth. We could live healthily, grow old gracefully and die healthily after a long and pain free life, perhaps. Or at least we could make the effort to aspire to do so.

Vegetables are relatively cheap and are highly nutritious. We need to eat for nutrition to make our bodies strong. Or at least we should do so. We do not need to eat for pleasure. Our bodies need the vitamins and minerals within foods to help them repair and grow. If we do not give our bodies the right and correct materials to build and repair, our bodies will start to break down in some way. Our bodies are like houses. If the house that you live in has slates or tiles that have fallen off, you buy new ones of good quality to repair the roof. It is the same with your body. The vitamins, minerals, calcium, and proteins that we take into our bodies daily are like new tiles and cement. They are the fabric of our bodies. They are the materials for repair and growth. An easy way to take the nutritional value of fruits and vegetables is to juice them. There are many good quality juicers out there on the market now. They are not as expensive as they used to be. To juice is an easy way of getting the job done. Drink your vegetables? Why not?

I suppose that at the end of the day good health is not rocket science. It comes down to individuals being mindful of their own situations and the nutritional necessities required by their own bodies. Eating too much of the wrong things all of the time is bad for us. I gave up depriving myself of the things that I like to eat years ago. It did not work for me. However, I do not eat chocolate every day or cakes every day. I eat them from time to time when I wish to. I am mindful on a daily basis of what my body's nutritional needs are. My body requires a variety of foods each and every day.

The way you think, the way you behave, the way you eat, can influence your life by 30 to 50 years.

—Deepak Chopra

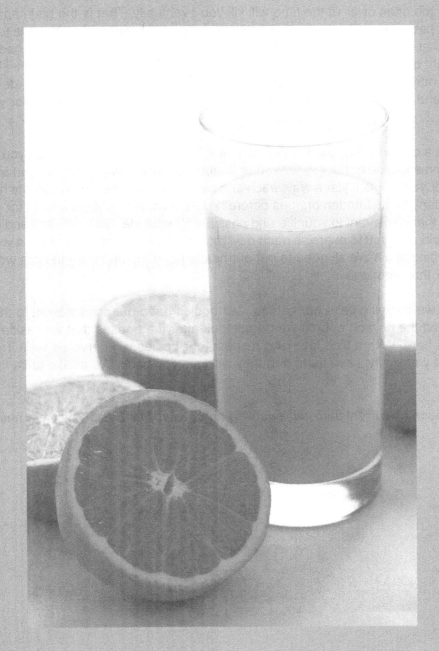

I suppose at the end of the day good health is not rocket science. It comes down to each individual being mindful of their own situation and the nutritional necessities required by their own bodies.

—Lynette Avis

My first port of call each day is to ask myself what it is that my body needs today. Do I need to eat more fruit today? Do I need to eat some fish today? Should I eat this or that today, as I have not had any this week? These are good questions to ask each day. A few simple questions on a daily basis go a long way. It is not good to eat the same foods all of the time, as our body needs to have variety. It needs to gain its nutrition from far and wide, so to speak. To eat beef burgers and chips every single day will not give your body all that it needs. To eat beef burgers and chips once a week or once every two weeks is very probably fine. A little of what you like keeps life sweet. Deprivation is not good for the soul.

Over-indulgence too often or all of the time will kill you eventually. That is the plain and simple truth of it. We each of us have one body. If we have the good fortune of having a healthy one to start with, then why not keep it that way for as long as possible? It does require a little effort. We need the right food choices in the right quantities, as well as the dreaded 'E' word—hands over the ears—EXERCISE! We all have to move our bodies. Move them, move them, move them . . . de, de . . . de, de . . .de dum! Put some music on and get on down to it, as they say. Make it fun. Whatever is fun for you, then that is what you do.

Do not do what is a chore to you; you will not stick at it. Find something that excites you and makes you feel good. Is it tennis for you or hockey for you or football for you or swimming for you or martial arts for you or dancing for you? Or is it just a walk each and every day with the dog or, as my husband does, a brisk walk over many of the London bridges before he gets into work? Make it work for you. Build it into your life in a way that is relevant to your life and possible for your life. Do a bit each and every day if you can. If it is impossible for you to exercise each day, then do it just two or three times a week. Something is better than nothing at all. We all need to get our hearts pumping and our muscles working. A little bit regularly is better than nothing.

This is a gift that we can all give to our bodies. Our bodies need our commitment to them. We cannot live in the here and the now on earth if we do not look after the houses that we reside in. I am talking about our bodies here. With a little love and respect, our bodies will serve us well. Treat them kindly and they will treat you kindly. Love them and they will love you back. We all like to be loved, and so do our bodies.

For more information on current thinking regarding health and well-being visit www.nhs.uk

We Say . . .

One's physical health is an important part of the body's energy system. The physical body and the spiritual body are interconnected and affect and influence each other. Sleep deprivation, stress and anxiety, under- eating, or over-eating, poor nutrition, over-exercise, and a lack of exercise all affect our physical being, our spiritual well-being, and our sense of energy.

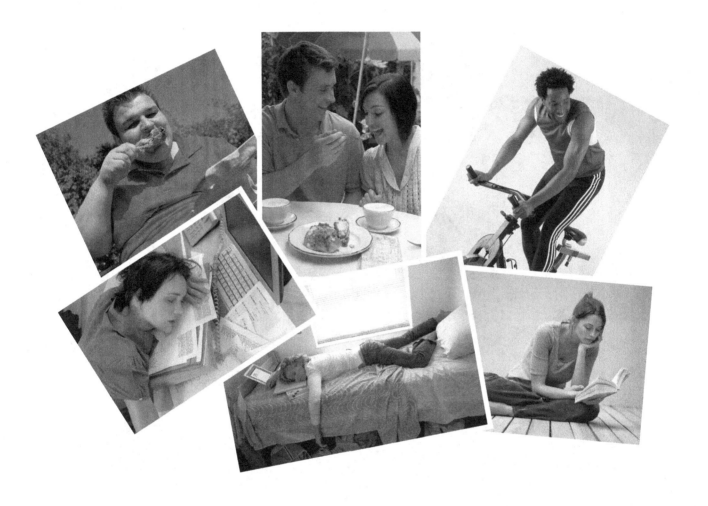

To keep the body in good health is a duty . . . otherwise we shall not be able to keep our mind strong and clear.

—Buddha

It takes more

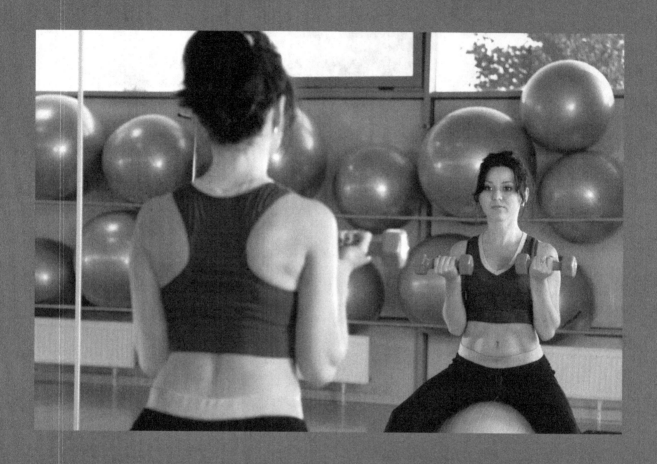

than just a good looking body. You've got to have the heart and soul to go with it.

—Epictetus

Be at Peace

How can we be at peace when life is often not at peace with us? Words are easily said. What is the alternative to being at peace? The alternative is to wage war on our fellow man or on ourselves. Whatever happens to you within your life has a reason. There will always be bad things that will pass your way as well as good things. It is not the bad that will come your way that you should worry about; how you respond to the bad is the most important consideration. Each action sets other actions in motion. In action you have power. In action you have the power of choice. There are billions of people who walk the earth.

Each person performs countless tasks each and every day. Each person makes many decisions each and every day. Each decision is a personal choice. With each one of those choices that are made and put into action, a flow occurs. A flow of energy is set in motion. We can set an action in motion that is not peaceful if we so choose. That action will pass onto the next person and have its impact. The outcome of that impact cannot be foreseen, but it can be surmised. If a person lives their life in a violent way either verbally or in violent action, then that is what is sent out to the rest of the world. That is how the world will judge that person. The world will see the person in a violent light and will deal with that person accordingly. A violent action will bring about a violent response from others.

Our days are a mixture of actions and responses. Our actions and responses are crucial to our lives and the lives of others. Each action or response sets in motion another action or response. We create the actions and we create the responses. It is ourselves alone that we can either chastise or pat on the back for any outcome to our actions and responses. Our words to each other are both equally actions and responses. A sentence spoken will set energy in motion to the person it is spoken to and to the wider world. A verbal response to that spoken sentence sets afoot another action. So it goes on. There is a never-ending stream of action and response. From the beginning of mankind it has been so. Take a look at any history book and look at the lives described. Were those lives not a succession of actions and responses? Some people won, some lost, and some lost their lives on the merits of their personal actions, inactions, and responses to whatever situations, actions, and responses were thrust upon them. Inaction is as much a response as action is. It is a choice. It is still action, in that it is action withheld.

Each and every morning we wake up to a brand new day. We do not wake up to entirely new actions and responses. We wake up to the situations that our previous actions and responses have delivered for the new day ahead. Within the new day, we indeed will set out into the wider world more actions as we think, move, decide, and act. This is the choice that each of us has each day. We can choose our personal actions and responses within any situation that is on our daily path.

There are billions of people in the world, and every day they all interact with each other. An action is set in motion on one side of the country or in the wider world, and that sends out a tide of action energy. This energy ripples through the community of humanity, touching each person in its path. Each person with whom the action has contact will have an impact, and each person will react to that impact with a response.

Every one of us is responsible for our actions and responses. We are responsible for what we send out into the world each day. None of us gets it right all of the time. That is part of the self-development that life offers us. We learn when we get it wrong, and we learn when we get it right. Life can be a daily struggle, and life can be a daily joy. Not everything that you will endure each day will be of your making. However, on some level you will have played your personal part. Each lesson learnt, each misery endured, each joyous encounter has a foot in your past. If you were to walk out of your house and encounter a situation that was to bring about your demise, it was you and you alone decided on the action. Even if someone asked you or told you to step outside, you decided to do so, and you did so. Your decision and action put you in the right or wrong place to receive the full consequence of your decision.

We all play a part in our own lives and those things that come in our direction. We are not in total control, it is true, as we do not choose all that comes in our direction. However, in most cases we do choose much of what comes into our life because we choose what we do in terms of our personal actions and responses. If others find our behaviour objectionable, then we can choose to change it. If others find our dress objectionable, we can choose to change it. If others find our manners lacking in our personal actions or responses to them, we can change them.

It is obvious that if we change those actions and responses that do not bring us the greatest good, we will change the energy of our lives. We will bring about improvement within our life, if indeed improvement is what we are requiring of the situation. What we can do on a personal level we can do on a global level. Equally, even on a global level all is action and response. The trouble is that on a global level it is far more difficult, as there are many more people creating action and responding to any given situation. Obviously this is the difficulty. To accommodate all is impossible, so we accommodate the majority. Maybe that is the best that we can achieve in these sorts of difficult situations.

The best each of us can do is to be mindful of the flow that we each set in motion each day. Be mindful that we do have power, however small and however insignificant we may feel it is. It is a power none the less. It is the power to manifest positive or negative through our personal choices in our actions and responses. We and we alone are responsible for the good or the bad that we send out into the world. If we act without clear thought and without a good and honest heart, we will endure the consequences of that. It is that simple. When you are at peace in your heart, then your body too is at peace and is in balance and harmony with all that there is. Energy flows, and you are in charge of the energy within your body and its flow out to the wider world. That flow is connected to the way you respond to the world and what you send out into the world also. To keep well, act well and respond well, and all will be well.

By three methods we may learn wisdom: First, by reflection, which is noblest; Second, by imitation, which is easiest; and Third by experience, which is the bitterest

—Confucius

We Say . . .

By accepting the things we have no control over, we are empowered to influence the things we do have control over and so develop as much control in our lives as we can. It means we can take responsibility for our lives and our actions. That in turn has an impact on all aspects of our lives including our health.

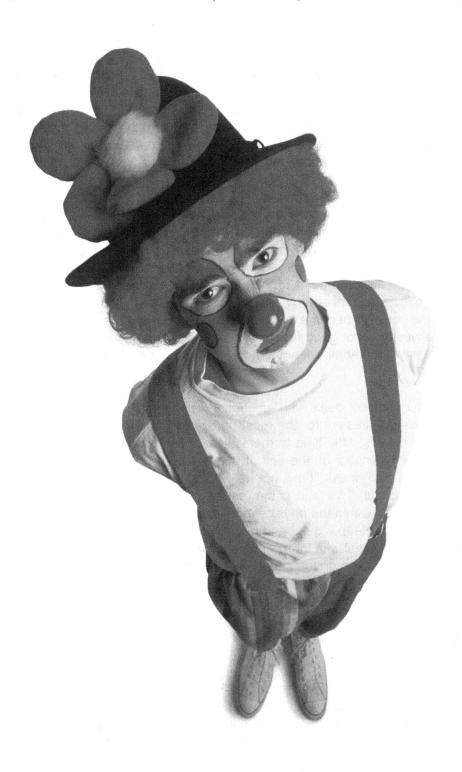

Set 2: Meditations for Health and Well-Being

Health Meditations Explained

These meditations are for people who wish to or need to improve their health. They are for the three areas of our physical health. Meditation has a great impact on the condition of our health. It will improve your health and well-being if you do the meditations regularly. That does not mean that you must meditate each and every day. What it does mean is that you should meditate a few times a week. Keep meditating going, just like you would ideally do with physical exercise. Sometimes it is not good for us to exercise vigorously each day, as the body needs a rest and time to recover. The body does not need time to recover from meditation, but you need some time to absorb the impact that meditation is having on your well-being and time to get used to the idea of making it part of your life routine. Take it slowly, and you will probably be more likely in the long term to stick with it. You know yourself better than I, so do what feels right for you.

The first meditation of this set deals with physical health directly, the second deals with emotional health directly, and the third deals with mental well-being. The physical well-being meditation works by rejuvenating and renewing the physical body. This meditation does this by expelling unwanted and stagnant energy from the body. Most often we hold onto stagnant energy within the solar plexus itself. Our emotions are released from the heart to the solar plexus. We need to expel any stagnant energy from this area of the body if stagnant energy has collected there. If stagnant energy has collected in this area for a long time, the body will become overloaded, and it will send the stagnant energy back around the body. Stagnant anything is not good for the physical body, and stagnant energy travelling around the body will not do it any good at all. Cleaning and renewal of energy always leads to rejuvenation of the body.

The second meditation of this set deals with emotional well-being. Stress is said by doctors to be the silent killer. Our lives are so stressful for the most part in our modern society. We all lead such busy lives, and many people have so little time to themselves these days. This constant doing and lack of rejuvenation has a negative impact on the self. It puts stress on the person and their emotions. It is said by holistic healers that all illness, if it is not hereditary, starts in the emotional body of the person first. Our emotions become out of sorts, and the result is that our physical body next becomes unwell as negativity becomes stored within the physical body over time. So to maintain good physical health, keep your emotions in check. Keep a quiet and harmonious outlook and demeanour. Do not let things make you overwrought. Try to deal with them with peace and quiet in your heart and being. The bottom line is this: if you have no influence on the situation, then let it be. Do not let it stress you, as the result will be damaging to your health. The less stress you feel when dealing with the situation, the more effective your input will be, as you will have clear thinking. So the second meditation of this set is the thing to do to cultivate the calm that you need to stay focused and quiet. In fact, do this exercise at least once a week. My co-author does this at night before he goes to sleep, he tells me. It is a good idea to do it when you are in bed, as it will take you off to sleep.

The third meditation of this set deals with mental well-being. This meditation is for everyone. Everyone needs a clean and clear mind. This meditation will help anyone who is suffering from a problematic mind. It will not necessarily cure their mental ill health; however, it will take them into stillness, calm, and peace. It will help them. For some people this meditation will be all they need. Others will still need the expertise of conventional medicine, depending on the condition that they are suffering from. If they have just little blues of the spirit, this will help to lift them. This meditation will help in some way, and it will be positively impactful even though it is not a cure for severe mental ill health. This meditation must be done every day if possible.

Meditation 1: Physical Health Meditation

1. Bring your awareness to the solar plexus.

2. Imagine there is a ball of energy in the solar plexus.

3. Grow the energy. Now send this energy down to the ground.

   Repeat this at least ten times.

Each time you send the energy to the earth inhale a breath and also bring clean fresh air into the lungs.

Meditation 2: Relaxation Meditation

1. Bring into the body energy through the crown of the head. As you bring the energy slowly down into the body, relax the body and awareness.

2. Imagine small particles of energy moving around your body, and as they move they gather tension and unwanted negativity.

3. Send the particles down the right side of your body first. Allow them to move slowly, and as they move, imagine they are sponges soaking all unwanted debris in the body.

4. Now take the energy into the right leg to the tip of your toes.

5. Now bring the energy up the right leg to the waist.

6. Now take the energy down the left leg, gathering negativity and debris as it travels.

7. Now bring energy back to the waist.

8. Now take the energy up to the solar plexus and expel the energy through the solar plexus.

9. Repeat from start to finish three to four times. Alternate each side of the body. First treat the right side and then the left.

10. Now you should feel lighter and cleansed. Take some deep breaths in and out. With each breath out, send out negativity and negative thoughts and emotions.

11. Now bring your awareness to your solar plexus and fill it with energy.

12. Now slowly send this energy around the body so that it travels one side of the body and then the other, returning to the solar plexus.

13. Allow the energy to circle the body two or three times.

14. Bring the energy back to the solar plexus, and just sit in this space. Allow yourself thirty minutes or as time allows.

15. Allow yourself to sink into total relaxation. Come back when ready to do so.

Meditation 3: Mental Well-Being Meditation

Bring the body into relaxation. Do this by taking deep breaths in and out slowly. This brings the body into relaxation. Allow all thoughts to float away. Let them go. Empty your mind and repeat these words.

Peace, quiet, stillness.

Peace, quiet, stillness.

Peace, quiet, stillness.

Take a deep breath in, and now slowly breathe out.

Peace, quiet, stillness.

Peace, quiet, stillness.

Peace, quiet, stillness.

Take a deep breath in, and now slowly breathe out.

Peace, quiet, stillness.

Peace, quiet, stillness.

Peace, quiet, stillness.

Repeat this many times.

Next do the same, but with the following words.

Calm, cleansing, clearing.

Calm, cleansing, clearing.

Calm, cleansing, clearing.

Take a deep breath in, and now slowly breathe out.

Once again, do this many times.

Repeat as above, but with the following words.

Empty mind, clear mind.

Empty mind, clear mind.

Empty mind, clear mind.

Take a deep breath in, and now slowly breathe out. Once again do this many times.

This will take your mind into stillness. It will clear and free your mind. This meditation must be repeated on a regular basis for maximum benefit.

Now focus on your breathing, and just bring your awareness to your body. Wiggle your toes. Focus on your feet, legs, etc. This will bring you back to the here and now.

Change your thoughts and change your world.

—Norman Vincent Peale

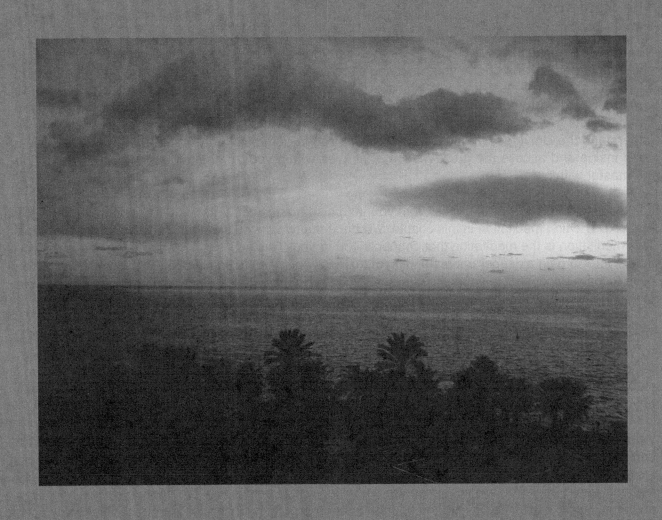

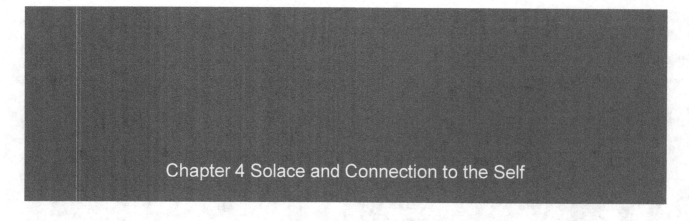

The Real You

So now we are getting to the crux of it– the real you! Until now, it has been about connecting to something greater, and I hope you have had success with it and have enjoyed the feeling of joining to something that is vast and yet intimate that cares about you, something that also wishes to impart its wisdom to you and share in its magnificence with you. Now we come to the part of you that connects to that greater part of the Universe and why you feel at home and at peace there. To understand the Universe, we must connect to it through going inwardly first and then outwardly. Go deep inside and access the great wisdom that lives within you. As the sages in the East said, find the master within.

It takes time and it takes trust. Trust *from* you, and also trust *in* you. First, you must come to know the real you. The first meditation in this chapter will bring the two of you together, perhaps for the first time. This meditation is the meditation that connects you to you. This you is the greater you. This is the you that is you. To gain a deeper understanding of this you, you need to first locate it within your being. You have to learn to connect to yourself. This is the you that is those gut feelings and instincts. It is the part of you that reacts when the road ahead is fearful or undisclosed.

To gain a deep understanding of the one that has always been there, the one that has always stood by your side, the one that wants to help and heal and love and hope and dream if only it was given the chance, you must go inside. You must learn to connect to that part of you and allow it to help you steer your course. This is not a part of you that you should be afraid of. This part of you is the best of you.

With this knowledge of the "real you" comes a sense of the understanding of your uniqueness. You begin to understand that you are special as everyone is special. You are no greater, and you are no lesser. For too long, perhaps, you have thought that you are not good enough or perhaps falsely thought that you were better. You are not either. We are all incredible beings with the capacity to live a fulfilling and imaginative existence beyond the boundaries of our perceived abilities. Embrace this reality now. The first meditation of this chapter will give you proof that you are more than you imagine you are—that you are more capable, more powerful, more beautiful, more passionate, more alive, more loving, more giving, and more wise than you ever dreamt you could be.

We are born dependent beings. We need love, support, food, shelter, and care from others to survive the early years. We need to be taught with wisdom and experience so that in time we become independent. Too often we grow into adulthood very much dependent on others. Our needs are fulfilled by others, as we cannot stand alone. We perhaps do not feel we have the inner resources to be able to handle the battles life has for us. We seek shelter under the wings of others because we feel incapable of facing the tide of pain and hardship that comes our way. Nothing could be further from the truth. You can discover this inner strength.

This first meditation of this chapter enables you to move past dependence into independence. The self within is the greater self. Why would you let you down? You would not if you truly knew the value you have.

Knowing Others

The second meditation introduces you to interdependence, the truth that you do not walk alone. To walk with others is to have their support, love, and strength, while you offer them your support, love, and strength in return. Together we are stronger than we are alone. A twig is weakest, a branch is stronger, but a bundle of branches is stronger still.

Know that all that you do affects all those with whom you walk.

We have a responsibility to others. The second meditation teaches us that responsibility. All that we think, do and say will have an impact not only on our own lives but also on the lives of others. We are all interconnected energetically, and we all have influence and impact. We are all absorbed with ourselves a great deal of the time. Most of us feel that we are the most important being to ourselves. We do not traverse life alone. We are social beings that cannot ultimately survive alone. We do have a responsibility towards other people. The human family is a family with which we are all interconnected both energetically and through humanity. We are not separate and we do not walk alone. All men and women are your brothers and sisters.

The first responsibility to yourself is to bring you in touch with yourself. The next responsibility that you have is to your human brothers and sisters, and the next is to the wider world. The second meditation teaches your responsibility towards other people. Without others, you live your life alone and in isolation.

Your Future, Our Future, the Future

This brings us to the third meditation of this chapter. Remember one of the great gifts that the Universe gives to man is "consciousness", or rather the ability to direct energy consciously. It means you have the power to shape your life and to mould your future into anything you want it to be. You choose your course moment by moment. That is all you have to do. That is all you have ever needed to do. In our naivety, we may think we are puppets at the end of strings controlled by other forces. We are not. We are independent forces that must live within a framework. We are interdependent forces that must work together to create a future worthy of our talents, passions, and aspirations.

We need then to learn a way of harnessing our gifts and directing the energy of nature towards a present and a future that has value and purpose. First we must gain a sense of our true selves, and then we can gain an understanding of our own power and connection.

Finally, we must appreciate the force of that connection and how it relates to the energy of nature all around us. This energy is not just in the present. It is in the past and the future. This is how we write our journey, and we must feel the path of that journey as we are writing it. To be in touch with the energy of our self and where it wants to flow is essential for life success. These three meditations make that possible. They bring into consciousness the power of your own being and the being of everyone and everything. They bring the sphere of influence you possess, simply by accessing the energy within you as it radiates into an ever-expanding present and into an ever-expanding future.

For too long I have lived my life on a day-to-day basis. There is value in that, but there is also potential missed that can only truly come from planning. But plan what? We try to bend life to our will. We try to make things happen by sheer force. We pray, we hope, we bargain with God, and some of it happens and some of it does not. Either way, we often feel exhausted at the end of it, as if we have fought against the current of some invisible tide or flowing river. It is as if we are fighting a natural flow, as if we are going against nature. The river is there whether you are aware of it or not. It flows with its great energy and power, in balance at all times, seeking the Way. If we fight this flow, we are out of harmony and out of balance, which means we are fighting to regain balance and harmony all the time. It is a constant struggle, and yet we are sure that we are pursuing the right path and that we have the right goals in mind and the means to achieve those goals.

"Free will" can come at a price, for there is a flow, and if we ignore that flow, we may feel at odds with a force and robbed of our power. There is a better way, a calmer way, a path in the flow of the river that may not be easier but that is far more exhilarating. We are not fighting the great current; instead we flow with it, and our "free will" has the chance to steer in the flow—right, left, or straight ahead. It brings with it challenges of its own, for it pushes us in directions that bear no regard for our comfort zones and our perceived strengths.

Instead we travel where we need to be next, leaving us open to new experiences and demands on our self that we may feel unsure of. We are forced to dig deep to find the answers within, to develop, grow, and evolve as we become the person we are meant to be. This is possibly a hard path, but it may be true that all paths have their difficulties. The key is that feeling of exhilaration—a little fear and apprehension for the unknown and the uncertainty, but a sense within that what you are encountering is right for you. You are on your path as others are on theirs. The meditations in this chapter help to develop your sensitivity to your journey and to the journey of others. They teach you to find your personal place within the world and to have respect for the place of others.

It requires a paradigm shift in thinking. No longer is it only about me and what I want. It becomes about what other people want as well. It is neither selfish or selfless, neither win-lose or lose-win, but rather win-win, when all sides to an interaction come away feeling they have achieved something worthwhile. We move forward together.

How do we know which way to go? This is when the energy "speaks" to us. You will come to recognise it over time, but it has a vibration to it, a feel that tells you this is the right direction. What may well follow is the feeling of fear or doubt that comes with realising that you are going to do something you have never done before or something that scares you. This is natural; it can be slowly overcome over a period of time. It is always there when you do something new. You start small and build up, and you gain in confidence and skill until this becomes your comfort zone and you no longer feel the fear. You have moved on and grown, and then it becomes time to work on the next challenge.

This direction that feels so right has many stages to it. You may not be sure exactly where it leads, but the direction and the immediate things that you have to tackle may be the right things to do at the moment. Or you may have a very clear idea of what the end result is, in which case you want to set out an action plan, a series of steps that may get you all the way or partially to your goal.

A lot of it depends on how far the goal is ahead of you. A twenty-year plan may be a little hazy. A two-year plan may well be crystal clear. Whatever the time frame, the journey ahead unravels like a man constantly walking towards the horizon. He can see three or four miles ahead, but he cannot see the whole journey, as the destination is on the far side of the horizon. He is aware of the immediate environment, what needs to be done now, and he is aware of what is up ahead. He can prepare and plan for the future, sure in the knowledge that he is paving the way for the future he feels is right for him. Changes, both subtle and drastic, can be made as required, always made with reference to the future and a sense of what feels right.

There is an energy and vitality to this path that revitalises you. The feeling that you are doing something worthwhile fills you with positivity, and this positive energy is infectious, rubbing off on the people around you and inspiring them to travel a similar road. Theirs is not your path, and the details of your journey are not necessarily theirs, but rather they travel their own way, a path that energises and revitalises them. We are all different. There is a path for everyone. We all have the chance to feel this vitality.

If only we could free our self of the bonds and shackles that limit us. Often put in our minds by others, these limiting beliefs are sustained by us, holding us back and making us think that we can only do this and that we cannot do that. Well-intentioned and perhaps not so well-intentioned teachers, parents, peers, siblings, and friends help us build a picture of our self that we can carry with us all our life. It means that we can go through our entire existence barely challenging any of these ideas, leaving our potential unexplored, untapped, and unfulfilled. If we can challenge these beliefs, the door to a whole new potentiality can open, and we can discover a whole new us that we did not realise was there.

This inner belief comes from within. It comes from a trust in the flow of the river of life and comes to those that "listen" to what is being "said" inside. It comes in the form of feeling energy. This is how it communicates to you—like a signal that is telling you you're doing it right. What we have to learn is to distinguish between the feeling of the energy and the feeling of the mind. The mind is limited by the beliefs that we have, whereas the energy is unlimited. It has built a Universe and has so much potential just waiting to be discovered. Will you listen, help, work, and overcome, or will you listen to words of doubt that hold you back and encourage you to fight the flow of the river? It sounds like a grand promise, but I promise these meditations point the way to the inner journey, a journey towards inner communication, towards inner peace and tranquillity, and towards inner trust of the energy within you that points the way to a life lived in harmony with the flow of life itself.

Sit quietly and still the room.

Still your body and your mind.

Now all there is,

Is energy.

That feeling is you,

The real you at this moment.

You are a silent bell ringing out,

Your vibrations touching the world.

What you feel now is you,

Not your clothes, your home, your car,

They are not you.

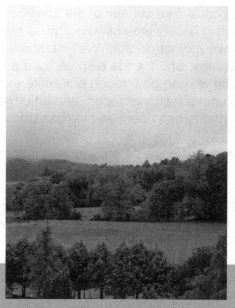

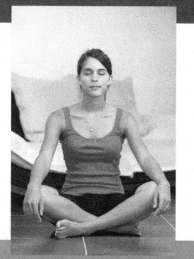

This feeling is.

It is the essence of your actions and your thoughts.

It is the essence of the way you see the world.

Touch this regularly and know it to be true.

Never allow yourself to be confused again.

You cannot stop the silent bell ringing.

Everyone hears it, so do not deny it.

Embrace it.

Express yourself fully.

You are already the vibration.

Do not be ashamed, and do not be shy.

This is you in your completeness.

Hide none of it. Explore all of it.

Honour it, cultivate it, and grow it.

Discover all that you can be and become,

And though sometimes the journey will be hard.

The journey will be fulfilling and you will do much.

This is all life is about,

Listening to your own bell

And to the bell of others.

It is the journey of truth.

David Brown

The Oneness of the Universe

The ancient peoples of the earth understood a fundamental truth about life. They understood that there were laws to life and its creation that governed their own lives. They understood that they were not separate from life but were indeed part of a greater whole. There is a fundamental law that governs the whole of life, and this is the law of mathematics and sacred proportioning. Sacred proportioning is a way of describing life and the systems of life throughout the universe. No part of that universal system is separate from each other. All life is an expression of the universal system.

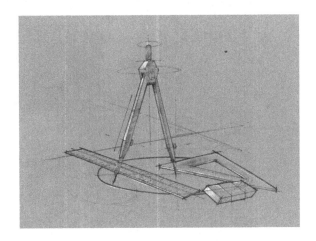

We can express that system of the universe through mathematical proportioning. The ancient peoples of the earth called that mathematical proportioning "sacred geometry". They used it to express the systems of the universe in a coherent and unified way. They used sacred geometry to try to make sense of the universe and the whole of life, life forms, and man's place within that universal system.

Modern science alludes to having all of the answers, but how can you ever do so if you exclude certain integral parts of that system in the quest for the unifying truth? Science excludes man's influence on the universe. Man is energy interacting with the energy of the universe.

Cosmology is the term used by philosophers to describe the entire self-contained universe and the human view of it. How humans view the universe is an interaction with it. Life interacts with life, and energy interacts with energy. This is a truth in life, energy, and the universe that man can be sure about.

Human beings are at peace when harmony is prevalent within the fabric of their being, their lives, and the wider community. Harmony brings peace. Sacred proportioning is harmonious itself because it expresses harmony. To view sacred proportioning brings about peace and harmony within the human condition, as well as expressing the systems of the universe and the harmony therein. The ancient peoples of the earth used sacred proportioning to express their understanding of the universe. They used it to construct great works of art in an attempt to recreate harmony and to express harmony and completeness. They did so to express the wholeness of the universe and the oneness of all things.

It is our intuitive attraction to harmony and harmonious proportion that often drives the human passion for science, art, and movement. When that perfection is clearly seen, heard, or understood, a feeling of power, a surging of energy, floods the being, and we are at peace. This is the beauty behind human life, the essence of all being.

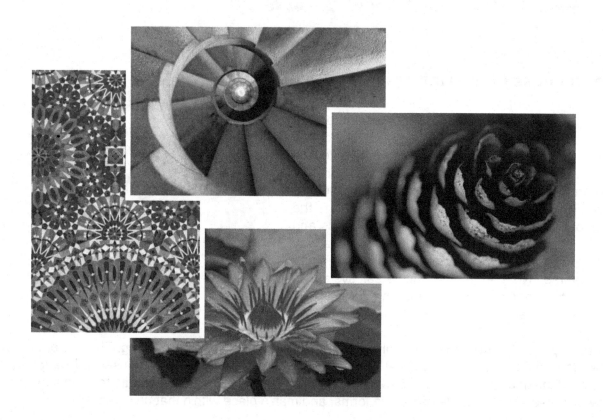

Life seeks perfect expression of form.

—Lynette Avis

Peace Comes from Within

As I sit in my conservatory and look at my garden and contemplate the word "peace", I would like to share some aspects of my life with you. I feel very thankful to be sitting here today and having this opportunity to talk about life. I know that I am a fortunate person to feel happy and at peace. I am at peace with all that is around me and that makes up my existence. It is not always easy to find that place of peace, and it eludes many of us for much of our lives. If we seek to have something that eludes us, then we will often find ourselves frustrated and unhappy.

When most people are asked what they wish for most in their life, they say peace. Where can they find peace in this life of chaos? We have only to look at TV or listen to the radio or read any newspaper to understand the level of chaos in modern life today. The world today is a dangerously troubled place. A person's life can be short or it can be long, and many days make up each of our lives. Within those days are many interactions with other people and situations. It is in those interactions with others and in those situations that we live our lives. We can all find peace if we know how to find it and where it is located. There are many ways to find this peace; the tool that this book gives for accessing the peace that so many of us cannot reach is meditation. I did not find the peace that I have now through meditation. Like so many of us, I went through many highs and lows to reach my personal place of calm. I lived my life with frustration and stress as I endured or reacted to what happened to me. Each of us has our own personal life story, and for the purpose of illustrating some points I have used my own.

At this moment my thoughts are of recent days in my life. I am thinking about three people who share my life with me —my son and two of my friends. My son came to stay with my husband and myself over the last few days, and of course it is nice to have one's son visit. That puts joy in any mother's heart. My son has been a troubled person; he is a young man who has been trying to find his way in life. He has still not found who he is or what he wants in life. As a mother, I look on and hope that one day he finds his personal peace.

Both of the dear friends that I speak of are at this time having to deal with the possible passing of dear and loved brothers. As a good friend, I try to make their difficult time easier. It is in painful or rough times that we need the help and support of others. We do not walk alone in this life, and we all need help from time to time. It does not matter how independent we think we are or how strong we think we are. There are always times when we need the love and support of our fellow man. It may be that there are good people around us to whom we can turn—dear friends or family—for that good advice or a friendly ear and a cup of tea. Sometimes in life we need a great deal more help than a cup of tea and a chat, but however severe the difficulty is, it is those people who care about us and whom we care about the most to whom we will most often turn to for help.

We do not walk life's path alone. However long or short our life is, we walk with others. We will each of us have many hardships to deal with in our life time. Difficulties come in many shapes and sizes, and they bring with them hard times more often than not. I indeed have had my fair share of life's difficulties. As I look out onto my beautiful garden and feel the warmth of the sun coming into the conservatory, it is hard to believe that the peace that I am enjoying on this particular day has not always been in my life. The condition of life is not fixed in stone. Our lives and indeed our perspectives on life change all of the time as we grow and as we develop as individuals. As we experience situations and conditions, they impact our thoughts and emotions, and we grow through them.

I am not sure if my life would be described by others as hard or not, though I do feel myself that I have endured quite a few hardships along the way. I have reached a place in my life where I have gained distance in both time and emotion from those difficult times that are now in my past. I do not look at any of the things that go to make up my life as negative, even though many negative things have come my way.

Everything that I have experienced along the way has brought me to this point in my life, and I am now happy and a wiser and stronger person for having experienced everything that has made me the person who has arrived at this point in time. That is not to say that I do not still from time to time have my moments when I look back and analyse my past. I do not think it is necessarily a bad thing to do that, because the ability to look back without anger or remorse shows growth of the person.

When I was in my teens, my father became bankrupt and my parents divorced. This was a painful time in my life, and life was a struggle for my family, as there was just not enough money to go around. My father had a business that eventually failed, and the family was left with lots of debts. We had enjoyed a comfortable life before that time. We were not rich by any means, but we had all that we needed in the way of food, clothing, and a decent roof above our heads. We lived in London and had many good friends around us. If I think back on those times, I suppose I could say that we had a hard dark struggle that followed a comfortable time. There were times when my family did not eat after my father lost his business. Those are cold and hungry times in my memory. This miserable period lasted about six years, but in fact it seemed longer. This was Britain in the days of the three-day week and the coal strikes. I remember that adding to the feeling of gloom.

My father decided to go to America after the failure of his business, and he found a job there. He was there for about two years, and our lives should have become easier. But in fact they became harder. My father sent us money, but it was not enough for the family, and my mother had to go out to work. My father had left some property to be handled by his solicitor. My father instructed this man to send the rent and any money from the property to my mother to keep us while my father worked abroad. To my knowledge, the solicitor did not do this, and I am not sure what happened to the money that was due my mother. I know that we did not see it as a family. Maybe it went to pay off some of my father's debts at that time. I do not know. I know this much: my mother, my sisters, and I suffered. It was a cold hungry struggle to buy what we needed to live.

I remember feeling so ashamed of our circumstances when my father lost his money. We had lived not a rich life but a decent and comfortable one. We lived in a nice home and had what we needed. Now there was of lack of the necessities of life. We struggled to keep our home and our possessions. It was all such a strain for a young person, and I remember becoming depressed and unhappy. This was the only time in my life that I have ever been depressed. I remember feeling isolated, ashamed, and alone. I tried to tell my mother how I felt, but she had her own struggles with money, and she eventually divorced my father. My father returned home after about two years and found work here. Very shortly after returning home—I suppose within five years or so—he lost his health and become very ill and nearly died. He lived for seven years beyond his illness and died at the age of sixty-four a broken, unhappy, and lonely man. When he was young he had a lot of friends, but many of them seemed to desert him when his life's fortunes took a negative turn. I would say that, apart from one person who gave my father help even in the last years, most of his friends disappeared.

I looked after my father for the last seven years of his life. My philosophy was that my father had always been a good father to me, and so I too would be good to him. This is what we all think will be the case should awful things happen to us, but the truth is that it is not always the case. When truly bad things happen to us, very often friends can be counted on one hand and with fingers a-plenty to spare. That is unfortunately the truth of it. However, sometimes we are blessed with the good fortune to meet life's gems. They are those people who cross our path and who make the biggest differences to us. These are the people who do take us in on a cold and rainy night, the ones whose very existence in this life make it a good place to be. True friends ask nothing of you but give to you. They enhance your life. We all hope to find good friends in life, but this does not happen for all of us.

I have an aunt and uncle who were such people to me. I did not know this when I was young, but they indeed did take me under their wing in their own way. When I was young, I resented in part these good intentions towards me. I do not know why. Maybe it was because they had such a happy life. My uncle was in the army, and my aunt worked in retail. Their children both went to good schools that my aunt and uncle worked very hard to pay for. By contrast, my family was scattered to the wind and thrown out into life. The breakup of my parents meant the breakup of my family. We all left home when our home was sold, and we all went to work, so there were no opportunities for us to go on to further education. We had to earn our own way in life, and so we all did. I think this was the resentment that I held, because I had wanted to go on to further education, bit I knew it would be impossible as I needed to put a roof over my head—and shortly after that, over my father's head as well. This I did throughout my twenties until my father died. Isn't it funny how often when people try to do their best by us, we still resent their help and good intentions? It all depends on our perspective and our understanding in a situation and life at any given time.

I am not a jealous person. I have never seen any wisdom in that emotion. I learnt at this time in my life not to be jealous, as it is a destructive emotion. Nothing happened to make me understand that. I just remember feeling those feelings once and hating them within myself. I decided never to have them again, and I never have since that time. This was part of my growth. Maybe I would have grown anyway and gained this understanding if this situation had not happened to me. How can I say?

I have three sisters, all of whom are younger than myself. I have always loved my sisters and have tried to do my very best by them. However, I do not think they have always loved me. I do not know if they have or even if they do now. Very often we do not tell people that we love them when we do. We just think that they should know. How will they know if we do not tell them? Maybe by the things that we do, that is true. By our actions we can convey many things. We can indeed silently convey love of all kinds. By contrast, we can also convey our hatred or our strong disapproval. How do we know that these silent messages are hitting the right spot? Well, for the most part we do not. We hope that they are. There is a silent connection that exists between all humans. We each of us have the power to talk to each other without saying anything. A conversation is always going on between us.

Each of us has our own agenda in life. Whatever that agenda may or may not be, we make our lives one day at time and so too our relationships. Relationships are made by two, for we have relationships with other people, not with ourselves alone. Sometimes we tolerate people because that makes our life and theirs easier. We say things like "let sleeping dogs lie" and "don't create waves". By this we mean that we should let things be and not stir things up. So by using those statements, we understand that we have the ability to take some sort of control within our relationships. People react to us all of the time. What we say and what we do and how we act matter. For it is in the way we behave that we win or lose with others. They will take offence or not depending on their point of view and on your point of view also. When our relationships go wrong, very often we blame the other person, but it is never the other person's fault alone. Whether we wish to acknowledge it or not, we have had a part in the breakdown of the relationship. A relationship takes two. It is the actions or non-actions that we contribute that will indeed impact in a positive or negative way. I am not saying that it is always the case that we did something deliberately to contribute to the breakdown, but on some level our behaviour and our actions will have contributed, for we will not have measured up to a mark in some way. Sometimes we will understand the mark that we need to reach, and other times we will not. It is there none the less, to our good or to our bad.

Some years ago my husband and I moved from London to the country like so many people do. We hoped for some peace and a new way of life away from the grey of the city. We needed to find a school where my son would be happy. I wished for some open spaces and a quiet peaceful life. I wanted to create a home that my family could enjoy—a home that would be welcoming to friends and family should they wish to visit us. I also hoped that we would make new friends and have many happy days in the country. For many of us that live or have lived in town moving to the country is a dream. My husband and I purchased a large property that was as dilapidated as anyone could imagine, and we set to work to make this wreck our dream home. We had a huge project and a smallish budget. For the first two years it was easy because we had a large lump sum of money to spend on the house. That money renovated a large proportion of the house, but by no means all of what needed to be done. There was a lot of sacrifice and a lot of hardship for us in the early years of living in that house.

There was a point where we ran out of money, and for years we could not do a thing to the house. We had a large mortgage, and each month there was no money to spare to do anything to the house. We could not save; each month we had just enough money to pay our bills and cover our basic needs.

My health at this time was very poor, and I suffered from ME, which came about once I started living in that house. I am not sure what caused my ME, but within the first year of living there I became very ill. I had suffered a viral infection that had resolved itself prior to moving, and I had been on the mend. My family and I had hard years in that house. I think if I look back on that time I can truly say that I did not enjoy one moment of living there. As a project it was exciting, and for an artist and designer there can be nothing much better than an interesting and challenging project. For me this should have been a time of great fun and enjoyment, but it was not.

Before we had even moved into our house and whilst we were in the process of purchasing it, the local people in the village decided they did not want us to buy that property. They did not know us, and so it was not personal. However, our house was their village pub and a house that had some local history. Obviously we knew that the property was a pub, but we did not know that it has the history and was a property that had some precious feeling attached to it by the local population. The house was estimated to be around four hundred and fifty years old. Just imagine the number of people who had passed through the doors of that house. Well some of the more recent ones had decided that we were not for them. We were upstarts from London and had to be excluded before we arrived. Our solicitor must have seen the unrest coming, because, unknown to my husband and me, he had secured a lock-out agreement on our behalf. This agreement meant that once we had agreed to buy at a price, no one else could put in a higher offer for the property and the owners were obliged to sell to us. Brilliant, my husband I thought—a stroke of genius on our solicitor's part! So within ten days of viewing the property we owned it. It was such a swift and smooth purchase the like of which, I am sure I will never be part of again.

We spent the summer with the help of builders making the property barely habitable, just enough so that we could move in and live on a building site. The house was very large, so we could live in part of the property whilst the other parts were being renovated. It all seemed so easy to achieve. However, within the first few weeks of moving into the property, I became very ill. During the first three months, I and my doctors thought that there was a real possibility that I might well die, I was so ill. The doctors were at a loss as to why I had become so ill; in fact, a few of them asked me that question. It was a question to which I had no answer to give. I did not know why. My poor health was to plague me for many years in that house, and I struggled to live and put that house together amongst poor health and lack of money and any support from people around me.

I do not expect strangers to help me. Most of us don't. When we have adverse times in our lives, we look to family and friends to help us. If they do not help us, at least we do not expect them to hurt or hinder us. Unfortunately, that is not always the case in life; there are many scenarios that are played out. Sometimes people react to situations because of a lack within themselves or their own lives. Sometimes when people see others seemingly obtaining the things that they personally desire and would have for themselves but cannot achieve; it is more than their hearts can stand. They often lash out at life and at those who have what they would wish to have.

This happened to me. My sisters, instead of being happy and excited for me, left my life and turned their backs on me. They left me to my illness and my large project in the country and only visited my house a very few times in all the years that we lived in that house. My family did not live very far from me—only about an hour or so drive away from where that house was. Even today many years later my sisters do not talk to me, having thrown me out of my own family. I am not invited to family gatherings anymore, and without going into too much detail, it was a hard and painful time for me. Maybe on a small level it still is.

There were, I suppose, some other underlying issues in the family and our relationships. However, the new house was the straw that broke our family relationship's back. So there I was in a large and (in time, and with much hard work and sacrifice) beautiful house. I had no friends because the village that I lived in mostly did not like my family or me. We had outsmarted them and purchased a property that the locals did not want to go to outsiders. My own family had turned their backs on me and my husband because we owned what they could not. My health was as poor as it could be, and if there was a time in my life when I needed help and a friend, then that was indeed it. If I look back on those times, I have no knowledge of how I survived. They were hard, cold, and lonely times for me and my family. It was all such a huge struggle, and we were all so desperately unhappy.

These difficulties that I speak of and have suffered are some of the things that go to make up my life. They are not things that, if I sat with pen and paper and asked what I wanted for myself, I would have volunteered for. If I were to do that—to sit with pen and paper and design my life—it would be very different indeed. I would choose for it to be happy, successful, peaceful, and fun, as most people would. Most people strive for these things in their lives, whatever else may be on their personal list of life's opportunities. How many people truly achieve them? Maybe some of us achieve them in part. Perhaps that is the truth for most of us. However, I do not think—and it is just my opinion—that many people manage to achieve happiness and peace all through their life without anything at all touching their lives or their emotions. Something on some level has to touch you or affect you somewhere. Life has challenges, and these are there to make us grow. They are the opportunities for us to step up to life's plate, the opportunity to roll our sleeves up and really see what we are truly made of. Some people seem to suffer more adversity in their lives than others. We all have our stories of good times too. I could also list my good times that were filled with sunshine. If I did this, I would be telling a different story. The one I have told you is the part of my life that was filled with dark clouds. There is an equal part of my life filled with pleasant memories and joy.

I have shared with you some of the difficulties that I have personally faced during my life. If you analyse the aspects of my life that I have shared here, what are they? We have had loss of wealth, family, and property, hunger, unhappiness, and desperation. We have had jealousy, struggle, rejection, pain, fear, ill health, and anger. Please go through the text and find for yourself what is there. It is all there. It is all part of life. All of these things make up life. In your life they will all be there also. You too will have your experience of some or all of these painful things. I know that there are many people who have suffered differently to me. Their sufferings may be harder or may be more acute than mine. If we look at other people across the globe, there is so much suffering out there in the world. Life is not a competition for who suffers the most. It is not a competition for who obtains the most good either. There are people who live their lives in this way, thinking that life is there for their personal taking and that it is a competition for storing up wealth, material or otherwise. Well, that is one way to live a life, but indeed there are many others.

All people live their lives in their own way, according to their location, circumstances, and desires. There is no right or wrong way to live any life. Getting solely what we wish for in life is not the truth of what life is. For at its heart, life is experience. It is the opportunity to experience many things. In our relationships we indeed experience much. With some people we will laugh and with others we will cry. In some of our relationships people will harm us, while in others people will bring us the greatest joys that we will treasure to the end of our days. Different people bring different gifts into our lives. We would not have a life if it was not for the interaction of others with us.

Imagine now that you live all alone on the earth. You are the last man or woman living here on the planet. No friends, family acquaintances, or strangers pass through your day—just you and the planet and no one else. Well, there may be those of you who are now thinking, "Goodness me, what bliss that would be!" I have to admit there are times in my life when that sort of peace would have been welcome. However, really think what that would mean. How old are you now? If we say that most people die between sixty and eighty, how many years would you have you to live alone? Think of all of those days that you will have to fend for yourself, not to mention talking to yourself. There is no one in life with you to help you with anything at all. What a struggle that would be and how miserable to endure forever. Maybe for a short time or some years it might be fine. But ultimately we are social beings, and we need the interaction of others. These interactions bring both pleasure and pain. That is the best of it, and that is the way it needs to be. There are challenges in life. How you choose to meet those challenges that life throws at you is your choice. There is no such thing as an easy life. Life can be hard.

My father said to me when I was very young, "Nothing lasts forever." This has been a statement that I have believed through life. It has been a statement that I have brought to mind in my own darkest hours. All things change and all things pass. However bad a situation may be, it is for *a time* and not for *all time*. It is best either to endure it or to embrace it. The choice is yours how you respond to what is happening to you. I promise you this, that there is always a lesson to be had from every situation. You merely have to look for the learning in each situation. It is hard to do this, I know. Even if the only thing you can learn is patience, then that is worth learning. When we are going through difficult issues in our life, perhaps the last thing we need is to hear that it is good for us. I have to say, though, that this is what I truly believe. It has been my experience of the things that I have had to experience. Some were painful at the time, but looking back now there is no pain, or very little. I have learnt the things that I needed to learn from them. I had to learn to let the pain go, and today I can pass on the knowledge to you.

Many people often perceive that money will exclude them from life's hardships. Is that the case, do you think? Let us examine this statement: "Money will bring happiness to me." If I go into any newsagents and look along the shelves, there will be a large assortment of newspapers and magazines. In amongst those newspapers and magazines will be those publications that deal with the lives of the rich and the famous. It seems that in the West, we have an insatiable appetite for knowledge of the goings on in the lives of the rich, powerful, and famous. I am not sure exactly why that is. However, in part it is probably that this knowledge adds some sort of spice to the everyday humdrum of ordinary lives. We often think that because we are ordinary people, our lives are humdrum. I am not sure that the rich and famous are any different to you or me. They too have their difficulties. If we think of the rich and famous, they too have their marriage break ups, affairs, and loss of face and favour due to poor judgment, miscalculation, and sometimes greed and selfishness. In short, it is all out there in life for each of us no matter where in life we may be. Kings and queens have lost their heads in the past, and history is littered with the rich, the powerful, and famous who lost out in the battle of life.

So if money, wealth, power, position, possessions, and family name cannot save you from the slings and arrows of life, what can? The truth is that nothing can. Life is life, and we are all touched by its adversities in some measure or other. Some bad or difficult things will come to you at some point. There will be things that challenge you, things that make you cry, things that give you pain, and things that make you want to throw in the towel and end the whole miserable affair of life. We are all equal in this in life. Life touches us all, and no one ever said it was going to be easy.

So if there are so many things in life that are there to make us miserable wrecks, why should any of us bother with this miserable affair that we call life? Why indeed? There have been times in my life when I have asked the same question. I think most people ask themselves that at some point. What is the point of going on? However I know this. When I was very ill, one of my doctors said to me that there was a possibility that I could not be made well I had become very ill. I looked out of my bedroom window just prior to Christmas and thought to myself that I might not be alive in the spring. I was so saddened by that possibility—not to see the spring arrive. I knew at that moment how precious life is and what a gift it is to each of us. I wanted to stay alive. I never thought about life in that way until I thought I might lose my opportunity to live here and now. I had always taken my life for granted, and I had always thought that I would be here until a ripe old age.

The truth is this that none of us knows how long life will last. As soon as we are born, the clock starts ticking. Time starts to run out as soon as we arrive here. None of us knows how long we have got. We just know that we are here now and that is all that there truly is. Today is the only true reality. Today is an opportunity for choice.

Today is in our own hands and no one else's. We have the power to live this day as we choose, or not as we also choose. In fact, everything is of our choosing. We choose if we stay alive; it is in our own hands whether we make the effort to survive this day. We have the power to make each day happy, for if bad things happen to us, we can choose how we deal with them and view them. We choose what we make of all of the things that happen to us. We can turn them to our advantage or not. We can embrace them or not. It is up to us what we do with the things that happen to us. In short, we make our own peace with our own lives. We make our own peace with the things that happen to us. We make our own peace with the people who cross our paths and maybe even cross us. That peace that we give out to the world and give to our own lives has to come from within ourselves. For if there is not calm on the inside, we will not display calm on the outside.

If bad things happen to us, and they will, we have the choice to meet them with a calm and quiet heart or to rant and rave. If you or I choose to rant and rave, what will that achieve? An early death or premature illness at best, I suggest. Stress does no one any good. To be continually stressed puts a strain on our emotions and on the emotions of those people who share our lives. It can impact our own health on some level or other. Therefore it is far better to try to maintain calm within oneself. I am not saying that it is easy. Very often it is not. However, it has to be said that calm people are nicer to be around. They are easy, like a breeze, just like fresh air to the soul. By contrast, people who are always angry or violent or distressed are no pleasure at all to be around. They are a danger to themselves and to others. They are not pleasant to know, as they are generally unpredictable and are a strain and a drain on our emotions, and that can have a negative impact on our health. Finding your own personal place of peace and calm is your choice, whether you do so or not.

Once again, notice those words "personal choice". You choose whether you wish to walk through life with peace in your heart or with violence and anger. It is your choice, for that is indeed what your life is—an opportunity to choose. Each and every day we make choices.

Today I chose to eat toast for breakfast and to sit in my conservatory and write this. I could have chosen to vacuum the house, but I thought, "No, I'll vacuum tomorrow or later perhaps." This was a small choice in life, I know, but it's a choice none the less. How we greet each and every day is up to ourselves. How we choose to greet the people with whom we share this life is up to us. How we choose to view the planet in which we live is up to us, and how we choose to view the negative and difficult things that will, as sure as eggs are eggs, happen to us is also up to us. We control our lives and the peace within our hearts. It is all up to us. Life often gives us bitter medicine for the soul; it can be very hard at certain times and in certain places. None of us gets things right all of the time. We are ever evolving and ever struggling. The fact that it is hard is not what we should concern ourselves with the most. It is how we greet each day that we live. It is how we live our lives and the perspective we take when we view each joy and adversity that comes our way. We are the only ones who can find our own personal peace. *True peace comes from within.*

Life is a country that the

Old have lived in.

Those who have to travel

through it can only learn the

way from them.

—Joseph Jouber

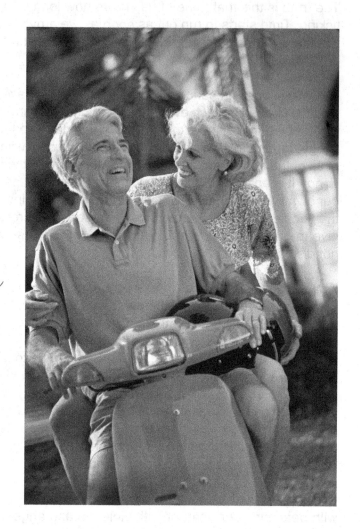

Life is either a daring adventure or nothing. To keep our faces towards change and behave like free spirits in the presence of fate is strength undefeatable.

—Hellen keller

We Say . . .

Peace comes from within. No matter what sadness and joy we experience in life, the source of how we deal with those experiences comes from within ourselves. How we brook disappointment, how we view success, how we respond to the things in life that do and do not go our way are manifestations of our inner being. As our life experience grows, we are encouraged to dig deeper into our self to find ways to grow and learn and move forward. This helps to make us self-aware. We have the qualities within to find answers to all the problems we face in our lives. Only by looking inward can we find a measure of peace within the hectic experience of our daily life.

We find a place of peace within that allows us to view the turmoil and joy in life with a sense that all will be well. For all will be well. All is as it should be. If we want change, we must look within and find a deeper part of our self that means that we change our view. It is called wisdom.

So much of our turmoil comes from trying to please other people, to obtain their approval. How can we be at peace if we seek to please everyone? We cannot please everyone! We are bound to disappoint someone and so face disillusion and frustration. So, rather than look outward at others for approval, look within instead. It is not that we should please ourselves without regard for others, however. Rather we should do what is right and true for ourselves. You must be true to yourself.

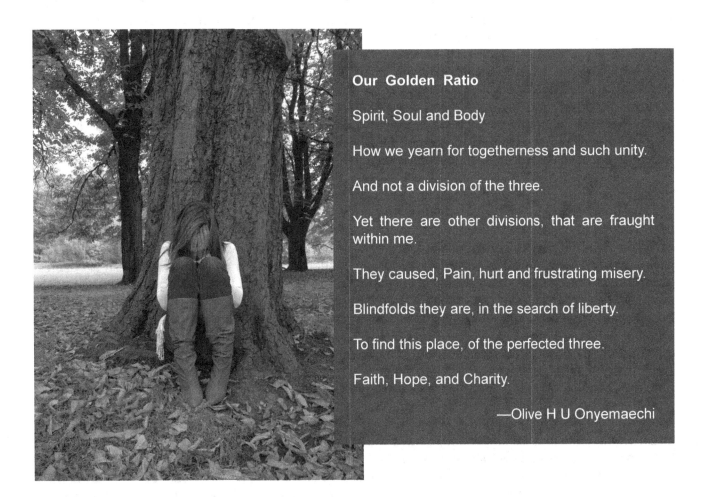

Our Golden Ratio

Spirit, Soul and Body

How we yearn for togetherness and such unity.

And not a division of the three.

Yet there are other divisions, that are fraught within me.

They caused, Pain, hurt and frustrating misery.

Blindfolds they are, in the search of liberty.

To find this place, of the perfected three.

Faith, Hope, and Charity.

—Olive H U Onyemaechi

97

Finding Inner Peace

We live a life that is full of disturbances of one sort or another. We have relationship disturbances, situation disturbances, work disturbances, and we have lif-in-general disturbances. Just living life and interacting with it can be a disturbance to our inner peace.

When we talk about inner peace, what exactly do we mean? We mean the calm that exists within our soul or our spiritual self. There is a natural calm that exists within that part of us. It is natural to our being to be in a calm state. Most people are not angry all of the time or hyper all of the time or frightened all of the time. Most of the time, most people are calm. It is when life throws challenges at us that we become frazzled. Our fight-or-flight mechanism comes into play. This mechanism is called by psychologists "acute stress response" and was first described by Walter Cannon in the 1920s as a theory that animals react to threats with a general discharge of the sympathetic nervous system.

We need this mechanism that exists within us to protect us. With some people it is switched on and stays on. They are in a constant state of readiness for something. This state of being is not good for the health. Being constantly in readiness for something threatening is taxing to our health.

Living in some urban situations can do this to us. There are certain urban situations that are a challenge to the human condition. We have all heard of the gang warfare that exists within certain places. Living in a situation that is cramped for space with many people in close proximity such as a city will often be taxing on the emotions, health, and well-being of the person. It is not surprising that in many Western cities, tensions often run high and spill over into violence. To feel crammed or hemmed in either physically or emotionally is distressing. I lived in London for a large portion of my life, and I always felt as if people were hemming me in. That whole feeling would make me feel very unwell sometimes, and I think that this had an effect on my emotional health, along with other factors. I lived in the suburbs of London, but even that made me feel surrounded and stifled. How much worse must it be for those people who live in poor housing and very deprived urban environments that are very densely populated? It is this cramped situation that often turns urban communities into what seems like a war zone. People become aggressive to each other, as each jostles for space both physical and emotional.

Sometimes urban places are the location of war zones themselves. To be living in this sort of situation will surely be distressing. I would imagine that anyone living in distressing urban situations such as these will be in constant excitement or fear. These situations are surely intolerable for anyone to live in. To be in fear of one's life in the place that one calls home can surely be nothing but miserable. This is how many people on earth live from day to day. It seems to me that to make an urban situation a war zone can be nothing but madness. However, if one's purpose is to kill a large number of people as quickly as possible, then that is the location that one should choose. No person on earth can ever be sure that the place that they call home will never be subjected to the ravages of war whilst we hold together the thread of peace with the threat of war. I do understand that this is a complex issue and that there are many political perspectives that bring about wars of all kinds. However, at the heart of this issue there is sheer madness. To kill one's fellow man is wasteful and nonsensical. What part of your humanity can you go to that finds the mechanism that makes this emptiness possible?

To live in poor housing and to have any sort of lack of adequate living standards will be a stress and a strain on the calm that we each need to have within us. To have to cope with poor housing or a lack of food and clothing or to cope with the loss of work and a lack of money to meet one's needs will bring about a disturbance to one's inner peace and calm. There are many disturbances that can bring a disconnection with our inner selves; there are many inhumanities that man inflicts on his fellow man. This is not new. It has existed within the human race almost as long as we have inhabited this planet, I am sure. Man has a capacity to exploit his own kind and to inflict all and any atrocities on his own kind at will, most often without thought or conscience. Too often he thinks in the short term and only of his own personal needs. He rarely looks at the bigger picture and what is set into motion as a result of his actions. If he does so, it will be to assess the outcome in favour of him personally and not the wider human race.

Few people have truly generous spirits or outlooks. We hurt each other under the umbrella of separate individual, separate country, separate people, and different gender. Most often our motives for anything are selfish. There is always someone above you and someone below you. Some people see this part of life the rich and the privileged demanding subservience from all of those below them. If you are at the top of the social pile, then almost everyone is below you. This may be the truth of it in part. However, as I said, there is always someone above and someone below. Big fish eats little fish. That is the way of this life. So we are all guilty at some level of selfishness and exploitation of someone else. Whatever we buy, consume, or use, exploitation of a person is very probably part of that thing's existence.

I do not think it is a natural way of being for man to be inhuman to his fellow man. None the less, that is what he does. If something belongs to you, why would you destroy it? Unfortunately, this is not a question that man asks himself too often. Man sees things in the short term. Man destroys or creates at will. Whatever suits him best in the moment at hand, that will do for now. Man is preoccupied with his personal well-being and survival, together with his personal gratification on all levels. He is not in the main concerned with who suffers as a result of his own comfort and well-being. Man does not always see his fellow men and women as companions to share life with. He most often sees his fellows as a tool to be exploited for his own personal gain. History is littered with the remnants of this truth. Unfortunately, man's exploitation of his own kind occurs on every level of society and in every situation. That is how life is. Generation after generation, man learns little. He repeats his mistakes or starts new ones afresh.

People have always talked of a "Garden of Eden" to retreat to away from the slings and arrows of life on earth. We all look for that elusive Garden of Eden, but somehow most of us do not find it. Life is harsh, and it is in part necessarily so. There is a part of life that needs to be harsh. Being hungry is harsh, and so it should be. If we did not have to find food each day to sustain our bodies and survive, then why would we move at all each day? We would not. We would just find a cosy pleasant spot and stay in that space. If we did that on a daily basis till the end of our lives, what would we gain? We would not grow as individuals, as people, or as families. Some of the harshness of life is necessary. Yet there is much of the harshness of life that is very much of our own making. Very often, we act selfishly with our own needs at hand, and then when the fruits of our labour are evident, we turn our backs and say, "Nothing to do with us".

Life is indeed harsh, but for every harshness that we endure or have endured, there are people right now somewhere in the world, who are enduring harsher circumstances and existences. Those harsh existences seem far removed from us; we are here and they are elsewhere. How can those harsh existences be of our making? We do not know these people, and we are not doing anything to these people. But we are. We are all interconnected within this life. We share this place called earth and all of its resources and in recent years we hear tell of how the earth is a smaller place. We travel from one side of the earth to the other in hours or days. We speak to people on the other side of the earth by phone or internet connection in real time. We send goods from one corner of the earth to the other at will. We all eat food and buy various goods, and trade is at the heart of all of our existences and survival. Trade is a necessary part of life for us all.

So where is the independence that we all feel that we have? There is none, not really. We are not independent one from the other. We all depend on each other at some level. We are one. We are indeed many, but we are one. There is not one of us that can exist alone in this life. No matter what we do, we interconnect with others of our human kind. That is life. That is the beauty of life.

This interconnection brings imbalances within life on earth. Life can never be truly balanced. We have seen how people who wish to address the unfairness that exists in our systems of organisation of wealth have often fallen and gone by the wayside. Life will never be truly fair. We are the same, but we have our differences at all levels of life. There is rich and there is poor in everything that we are or do. Nothing is static. There is difference and there is change.

In some ways, for me, this is a truly depressing picture of life. Let's face it, what I am talking about here is deprivation, greed, exploitation, hunger, war, famine, and all of the nastiness and atrocities of man. This is indeed heavy stuff, but how does it relate to this book?

Well we are one and we are also many. Now I do not just mean that you are one. You are one, this is true. You are you, and you are an individual. But there is much more to this than just you the individual. You are one in the fact that you are an individual human being. However, you are related to all other human beings also, whether you want to be or not. No matter who the human beings are, you have a relationship to them in their humanness. You are of the human family. So often we see others as outside of ourselves. You are of the same kind, the same pattern, and the same mould. Look to the universe for the truth of this.

"Other races are different to us." They may well have their differences to us—different customs, different hair colour, different skin colour, different beliefs and religions, and so on. Do any of those things make us all different though? I know that things have changed somewhat on the question of racial harmony. I know that there is political correctness now. Sometimes I wonder how much we have changed, and are things truly better on this score? I am of mixed race, and I still from time to time come up against other people's prejudices towards my colour. I was born to a white English mother and a black West Indian father in the mid-fifties. Things were very bad in those days for my parents and indeed for my sisters and me as we grew up. We were all in no doubt that we were not wanted by society. I still come up against this sort of exclusion even now fifty-five years later, and sometimes in the most unlikely of places. So it makes me wonder how far we have come.

My father had a theory about colour prejudice. He said when a person mentions colour to you and says how much they are not colour-prejudiced, then they are. For if they were not, they would not see your colour; they would just see you. They would see the human being and not the shell or the social, religious, or economic differences that may divide you. I think he may have had a point. Whenever I come up against anyone who mentions my colour to me as if I do not know I am not white, I think of my father's theory. There are differences between us all, as I have stated. To name a few, there are social, religious, economic, and location differences, and there are differences in our own bodies and traditions. For those superficial differences are the petty things that really divide us all. We are one race: we are a race of human people.

We allow these things to divide us so often. I could not care less about the hair colour or the skin colour of a person, their race or religion, or anything else that may make them superficially different to me. I know that others have social differences and traditional differences and religious differences and racial differences, and thank goodness for that! What would there be out there to excite us if we were all clones of each other? All of the human race the same and all thinking the same? Oh my giddy aunt, oh no! Just thinking about that sends my head into a spin, and my personal calm has left me.

One of the things that I liked about the family that I grew up in was that it was truly multinational. My aunt Sylvie said once that her family (our family) was all nations. For indeed the tradition of inter-nation marriage was continued beyond our parents. We have all sorts in my family. We have blue eyes, blond hair, brown hair, black hair, white skin, black skin, brown skin, and I could go on. Who worries about that in our family?

When I was a little girl in the sixties I used to look at my father and my mother and try to see how they were different. The racial prejudice at that time in Britain was acute. Racial messages came at me daily from the media and in my own general life. I tried so hard to see how my father was a lesser person than my mother because of his skin colour, and I just could not see it. It did not make any sense to me.

We are all the same. We all have our daily needs, and those needs have to be met. We cannot live without our basic needs being met. We have to eat each and every day. We need to drink water each and every day. We need to have clothing and shelter to protect our bodies each and every day. These are the basic needs of man. All men and women deserve to have these basic needs met. How we do that nationally or globally is the big question. Maybe it will never be achieved for all people everywhere at any one time.

This is a question for our world leaders. We are all selfish to each other on a global level as well as on personal levels, and we are selfish to our beautiful planet also. We are causing our own planet to heat up, but we still sleep soundly every night. Once again, has man learnt nothing? It seems not, I think. I don't think that any one of us is more or less guilty than the other. We are all guilty of abuse and neglect of each other and of our planet at some level and to some degree at some point in our lives. Maybe some of us try to move on and do better and live less selfish lives. I would like to ask you how easy it is to be totally selfless. Our lives are not solely in our own personal hands. We are all interdependent. This is the truth. A thought here becomes a decision there. An action here becomes a reaction there. Our personal daily existence sends ripples of thoughts, actions, and reactions out into the wider world. Everything that we personally think, do, or say leaves a mark on the world. All is energy or an energy encounter.

So now, with all of this madness going on in the world around us, how much inner peace can any of us have? We as a race, "the human race", "the human family", hate each other or dislike each other or are dissatisfied with each other for the most part. We have no regard for the earth home in which we live. We wreck it. Each and every day we are destroying this beautiful place we all share called "earth". How can any of us have any inner peace?

Maybe the starting point to all of this is to find the inner peace that exists within you. Maybe the road to inner peace it is to find that place of tranquillity that is somewhere inside of you. I know this much: if any of us truly thinks too closely about the truth of what we are doing, we would probably not want to go on another moment. For if mankind continues in this vein of selfish indulgence, he will then destroy what is most precious to him.

Somewhere, somehow there has to be change. For us to survive this time and this place and what we are all doing, there has to be change. That change needs to start with one—this one, you one, you. Each of us can only change ourselves. We are the canvas upon which we can draw. We can each individually be in charge of the energy that we send out into the wider world. Our organised systems of living are of our collective invention, and we all sustain them on a daily basis. We can each mould our own thoughts and beliefs, but we may not necessarily be able to persuade others that change needs to take place. If you want any change personally or globally, start with yourself and let the rest happen.

Be at peace within yourself first, and the world will be at peace with you.

Be You

We are not a sum total of our history, for we each have infinite potential. Along the way in life, you may have had encounters with people who would crush that infinite potential for selfish reasons of their own. Every so often in life, we meet these weak people, for that is indeed what and who they are. They will tell you that you have no talent, ability, or inner light. Know this: they are wrong. You have everything that they possess and more. It is just that you have not found that place within yourself where that light resides. Our history does not define us. Our history is a record of who we were yesterday. Yesterday is history. It is gone and will never return again. Today is the present. It is a gift to you, and you must embrace that gift and give thanks to life itself for allowing you this present day and all it brings in your direction.

Yesterday's lessons exist in your mind and in the fabric of your being. What you choose to do with the knowledge gained from those lessons is entirely up to you. If you had a bad parent, resolve to learn from their misdeeds or poor choices. Be a brilliant parent yourself. Do not complain about the school that life sent you to. Use it to mould you. That was the purpose of the school to which you were sent. Learn the lessons on a daily basis and slowly fashion the "you" that you truly wish to be and deserve to be. You are everyone's equal, no matter to whom you were born or where you were born in this life. The only person who can make you believe otherwise is you.

You have your own gifts and talents. You bring your uniqueness to this world. What you choose to do with that uniqueness is up to you. Fashioning a beautiful work of art takes commitment, time, persistence, thought, understanding, and will. You are a work of art. There is no other like you anywhere on earth. You are as unique as anyone can possibly be.

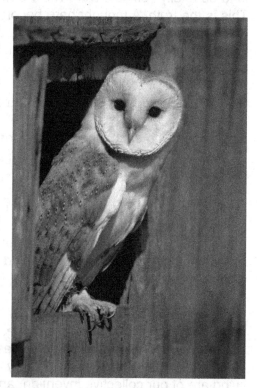

Work hard, read many books, and absorb knowledge and good information from true and decent sources. Observe life for life. Observation is its own teacher. It is its own school. Take wisdom from wherever you can find it, and be generous of spirit and pass that wisdom on to your fellow man. You are all you ever have to be. *Just be you.*

Every time you don't follow your inner guidance, you feel a loss of energy, loss of power, a sense of spiritual deadness.

—Shakti Gawain

If you judge people, you have no time to love them.

—Mother Teresa

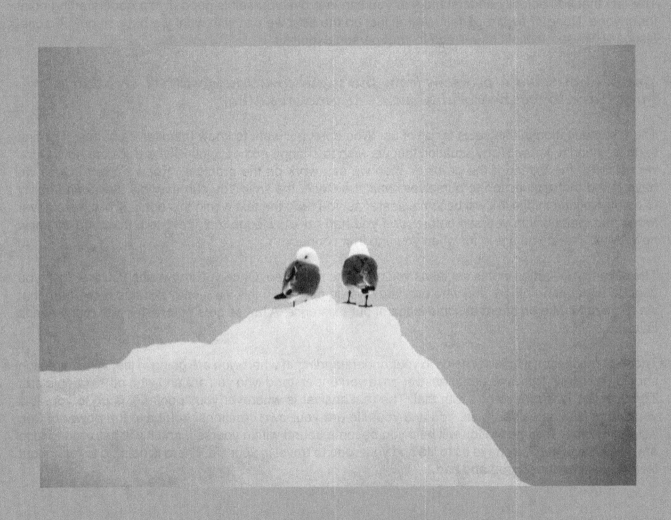

Self-Growth and Life Awareness Meditations Explained

These meditations are for self-growth and life awareness. There are hundreds and thousands of books written on this subject. Some of those books are excellent. These days we have become much more aware of ourselves and of our own corner of life. We are being encouraged to see the self as a work to be honed more and more. Maybe it was always that way, and we are now just coming at the problem from a different angle. In the past people would look to the established churches to help them discover themselves and their role and place within the cosmos. I can see nothing wrong with either approach. The fact that you actually understand that you can improve yourself is good. It is a good starting point for anyone. None of us are perfect. We all just do the best we can with what we have at our personal disposal. These meditations will add to your personal took kit.

You cannot solve a problem from the same consciousness that created it. You must learn to see the world anew. —Unknown author

The first meditation in this set is for all of us. Who does not want to know themselves better? The first thing we need to know in any situation that we wish to change and develop is where we are now. Once we establish the extent of the problem, then we can work on the problem. "Know thyself." Once we have found that connection to ourselves, well, the sky is the limit. You can use this new-found ability to do marvellous things. All will become clearer as you read the text within this book. If you have never found that place within yourself before, or if you had no knowledge that it existed, then you do know now. What a treat you are in for when you find that connection.

The second meditation in this set takes you on to the next step. Once you know who you are, then you need to understand others and who they are. We do not live in this life alone, and this is the truth that we all need to take on board at some stage of our existence. A house gets built faster with many hands involved.

The third meditation in this set helps in your understanding of where you are going in life. What direction should you take? This is easier to answer once you understand who you are and who other people are. The question is where you go with that. The real answer is wherever you choose. It is up to you. It is your life to fashion as you wish. You and your life are your own creations. You have the power of free will and choice. This meditation will help you become sound within yourself, and it will help you to lose any fearfulness you may have as to life and your road to travel in your life. There is nothing to fear about life. All is experience, good and bad.

1. Bring yourself down into relaxation. Bring yourself to a place of calm and relaxation.

2. Take many deep breaths. This is very important. One needs to oxygenate the body to gain the necessary degree of relaxation.

3. Count the breaths from one to twenty slowly. Then on the twenty-first breath, hold the air in for four counts.

4. Do this twenty to forty times as feels right for you. This will take the body into a very deep and lasting relaxation.

5. Next, take your attention to the solar plexus. Imagine that you are letting energy slowly seep out from this area.

6. As the energy seeps out, you become one with your own spirit. Feel the oneness of the self.

7. Gradually you should feel more and more connected to the real you.

8. Ask yourself whatever you want. Tell yourself whatever you want. You will be in the best space to receive what is needed from the conscious to the subconscious you.

   Feel the beauty of you. Feel how special you are, though not separate. This is the true you. Now let you slowly go and come back to the conscious you.

Meditation 2: Connecting into Others and Knowing their Needs

1. Take yourself down into relaxation. Now take many shallow slow breaths.
   Concentrate on the rhythm of your breathing. Know your own breath pattern. Listen to the rhythm of your own breath. Feel the calmness feel the beauty of each breath.
   Know you are an individual.
   Know that you are not separate.
   Know that you have connection to others of your kind.
   You are human and of the human kind.
   Know that you have brothers.
   Know that you have sisters.
   Know that you are one of many.
   Know that you are not alone.

2. Now bring white light energy into your body. Bring in the source. Ask for the hand of God to guide you. Connect to all that there is. Send out the vibration of healing. Know that it is in your power to do so. Send out to your brothers and sisters. Understand their needs.
   As they hurt, so do you.
   As they bleed, so do you.
   Send out the ray of compassion; send out the ray of love.
   Bring your attention to your own body. Now connect your spirit to others.
   Understand that you are one of many.
   Understand that you are connected at source.
   This is universal law. This is universal truth
   Now send out the vibration of connection. You know this connection on a soul level. Send it out, and stay aware and connected. Walk with your brothers as one.
   From this moment on, understand all that is.
   Understand you bleed as they do.
   Understand you are one of many and walk together as one.

3. Now feel the thread of connection and hold in that place for ten minutes.
   Now let the connection slowly diminish. However, always hold this knowledge. This meditation changes you for all time.
   Come back to the here and now.

Meditation 3: Knowing Your Future

Step 1: Start the recording by giving instruction on preparation, here:

Please refer to the section of Chapter 2 entitled "The Recording step" 1.

Step 2: The breathing pattern here:

Step 3: Lines to record below:

1. Connect into the solar plexus on a conscious level by bringing your awareness to that part of your body.

2. Now contemplate this part of your body and feel it.

3. Now take in energy through your crown chakra.

4. Send the energy to the solar plexus and back up the body to the third eye. Do this many times to energise the third eye.

   Tip: This practise should be done many times a day to energise this area. Do this for thirty days. On the thirty-first day repeat steps 1-4. However, this time ask a question of the future you.

Lines to record continued:

5. Your future is not fixed. Nothing is fixed. All is flexible. All is malleable. You hold the key to your future. You have outcomes. You have future lines.

6. The line you follow is your choice. Know that it is always chooseable and changeable. You do the choosing and you do the changing.

7. To change your future, send out the vibration of choice.

8. This is a strong vibration. Send it out with conviction. Conviction is strength of character. Conviction is the key to success.

9. Nothing in time is fixed.

10. Send out the energy of work. Your work!

11. Send out the energy of knowledge. Your knowledge!

12. Undertake to change.

13. Know that it takes energy. Your energy! Take many deep breaths, and picture your future. Decide what you want and know it is your right. You are equally entitled. You are equally special. You have every right to be you. Hold that thought.

14. Bring your awareness back to the present. Let the future take its decided path.

Step 4: Bring yourself back to the here and the now here on the recording.

Please refer to the section of Chapter 2 entitled "The Recording step 4".

I know for sure what we dwell on is who we become.

—Oprah Winfrey

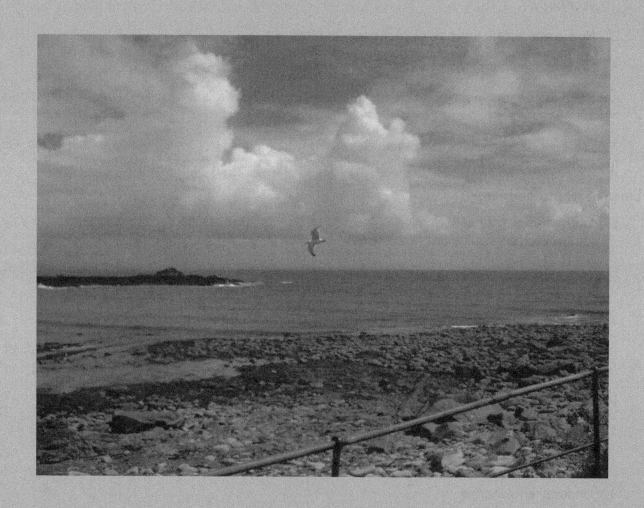

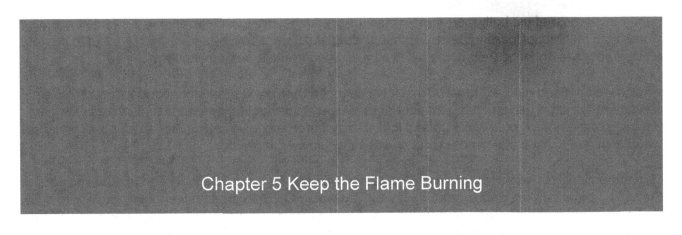

Voice, Uniqueness, and Calm

Keeping the flame burning is easier said than done. Each of us can only be ourselves, and yet how many of us aspire to being us? We look at glossy magazines and posters and advertisements, and we dream of a smaller us, a richer us, a better looking us, and a wiser us. We find constant fault with ourselves and feel like everyone else has it better than we do. The woman down the road has a better figure than us, and the man down the road has a bigger car than us, more expensive with plusher upholstery. There is always something about us to be dissatisfied with. Even if we go way back in our lives, there was always something to be dissatisfied about even then. Everyone else in the class at school was more popular than us and had better exam results than us and had who knows what more than us.

In fact, the whole going back in our-lives thing is best to be avoided, as most of us find that all of our dreams and illusions have been shattered along the way. Well, let's face it, how many of us have really got what we set out to have or achieve? No, best not look back and think too closely, as it is all a mess of shattered illusions and hopes and dreams. Of course we would all have done better at life if we had better opportunities, better friends, and better spouses—not to mention better parents and families. It would have been so much better if the right conditions had ensued and we had everything about us and in our lives in correct and perfect proportion. We would have been such better people, and such wonderful lives would have been the result. It is all so obvious, and it all stands to reason. This view has to be correct, because we are not bad people and we are not silly people. Our lives do not move in the right way. Everything about us and our lives is wrong. Every aspect of us is wrong, and so our lives are wrong. The messages that we are reading and viewing in the media and advertising are supporting our view of ourselves. We are told to buy this and buy that, and we will be instantly what we wish to be. Better skin, better looks, and better bodies will mean more money in the long run and happier lives. We all know this, because we are told this constantly.

We all have to look perfect, and if we don't, then we have to feel dissatisfied and give ourselves a good old beating up about our lack. Or if we do not give ourselves a good old beating, then we have to go to extremes in sorting out our lack of perfect looks. We need an expensive and risky operation or at the very least to add some goo into our bodies, silicone or Botox, to encourage the illusion of perfection. That will surely do the trick!

Of course there is no reason to look for any good in ourselves, because if our waist size is not minute and we do not have perfect looks and bodies, then nothing else about ourselves will possibly be good enough. We have failed at the first hurdle in life, so why think there will be anything else to feel good about? We all stand in front of mirrors daily and check ourselves out, and we always fall short of what we would like ourselves to be. We stand on scales and despair at the number each and every day, especially as it seems that the number keeps going in the wrong direction. It's all pain, misery, and more pain. I think most of us, both men and women, can relate to what I am saying here. Women are a bit worse than men about looks and perfection, but not that different. We see many men going into surgery for operations to enhance their bodies. It is all a growing trend in modern society.

What if we changed our view point? What if we changed the way we thought about perfection? What if we did not fall short each day and thought of ourselves as perfect? How would that change our lives? If for just one day you could wake up and look in that mirror and just feel happier about being you, how would that feel? I think that maybe relief and calm would be the result.

I have mentioned in earlier chapters that I suffered with ME for many years. Within about two years of falling ill, I put on an enormous amount of weight. I was a UK size ten and went fairly quickly to a UK size eighteen. I was size small, and then it felt like I was a size whale. All of my life I had been a small person, and that was how I thought I would always be. When I looked at myself in the mirror, a person that I did not recognise looked back at me. I could not exercise in those days, as my health was so poor and any physical activity would make me feel more unwell and my health would deteriorate. I had to resign myself to being a whale, as there was nothing to do about it for a while. When my health became a little better, I set about exercising, and over the years my size has reduced. I have not achieved the size ten that I once was, but I am now a little more realistic, as I am fifteen years older, and I have now settled on a size fourteen. Size and weight is not everything. It is not good for one's health to be oversized, and I am not telling you anything that you do not already know. Looks, good or otherwise, are equally not all-important for the success or well-being of your life. We can all look in directions other than our own and compare ourselves to others, and we will always fall short. There are in all things people who are better than us and people who are worse than us.

If we continually look at the situations of other people who we feel are better than ourselves in one or other area of life or being, then we will only make ourselves desperately unhappy. There are all conditions in the world. There are many people in the world, and each and every one is different to the next. All have some similarities but all are individuals and all are perfect in their own way. The perfection that each individual holds is the fact that they are unique. All that makes them is held only within themselves and no one else. There may well be others who look, feel, dress, express like you and seem similar. However, they are not the same as you. They can never be you. Only you have the power to be you. Only you have the right to be you. You are a unique creation. You are a unique expression of human life. No one will think the same as you, even though they may well be similar in how they think. No one will look the exact same as you, even though they could look similar to you. If you add those two things together—looks and thought—how many people do you think you could find who would have the same as you in the same way as you and in the same quantity as you? Now, you know and I know it is not likely that you would find even one let alone a whole bunch of people the same as you. If we start to add other factors into the mix, such as life experiences, interactions, and friendships it takes us further into uniqueness.

We all know that if we each of us were an art object, we would be considered a wondrous thing for our perfection and uniqueness. We are perfect, because we cannot be anyone else but us. We can only add to our perfection each and every day with our daily experiences. These are the things that shape us on a daily basis. These are the things that will add to our personal perfection.

Perfection cannot be found in the human body; if you look there for your personal sense of perfection, you are doomed to disaster. When we are young, strong, fit, clear skinned, and toned, then, yes, we may be able to smile at what we see looking back at us in the mirror. Look in that mirror every day from youth into old age, and see how dissatisfied you will become in time become. Make that inspection a daily routine throughout your life, and feel the sadness that will in time creep in. It may take longer for some than others, but our bodies are designed to disintegrate over time. Our bodies are like beautiful flowers that break through the soil slowly to unfold their perfect form. Once that perfect form has blossomed, it is there for us all to share for a time only. It then slowly says goodbye and then withers and dies. This is the way of all life, including human life. We are no different. We can only be the best we can be in this particular moment, as in all areas of our life. Our physical form is subject to the laws of life on earth. We are born, grow, wither, and die. Sorry if this is new news to you. I think something inside of you tells you that this is the truth of it. We cannot defy the laws of nature; we have to bend to her grace and wisdom. Mother Nature knows best. So now you understand that the ravages of time will indeed catch up with you sooner or later, perhaps mentally you would rather live with your head in the sand. Well, that of course is a choice. But maybe it is not a good one or the best one.

The thing that each of us must understand about ourselves is that we are a part of the process of life. We are life and part of life. In the time that we live, we bring good to life as we bring our unique selves to the mix of life. Just by being here each and every day, each of us changes something for the good or the bad. In everything we say and in every interaction we have with other people, we add to life. It does not matter how trivial the interaction is or how profound it is; we add to life's complexity and multi-layering. We add to life daily. If we say yes to something or someone, we add to life, and if we say no, we equally add to life. If we embrace something or reject something or if we say hello to something, we also add. Everything we feel, do, or say will add to the beauty of life. You are a creator of life's tapestry. You add to the painting each and every day. When you are grumpy, you are adding, and when you are sad, you are adding, and when you are happy, you are adding to life here on earth.

You bring to life all that you know, all that you understand, and all that you have yet to know and understand. You bring your unique potential. Life needs you and you need life, for it is by that interaction of life with you and you with life that the earth thrives or fails. There is a lot that rests on your precious shoulders, for life is not to be taken for granted. All that you are and all that you do matter, because you matter to life.

You do not have to do something great to be a great person. You are already great. You are you, and how wonderful is that? You do not have to stand under anyone's umbrella; you have your own. You do not have to walk away from anyone's light; you are your own powerful light. You do not have to share anyone else's light; you shine brightly enough yourself.

Understand the power of being you.

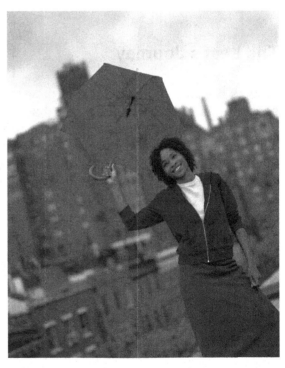

We Say . . .

To keep the flame burning within is a great skill, a great art. There are so many distractions that lead us to chase false rainbows. Part of the skill is being able to work out what is right for us, what is true for us. There is always someone ahead of us in the rat race, always someone behind, and we can spend our lives running from the people behind us and trying to chase the people ahead. We think this is what we want, but it is a journey fraught with worry and anxiety, for our sense of contentment is dependent upon our position in the race.

What if we changed our viewpoint? What if we changed the way we thought about perfection? What if we did not fall short each day and we were perfect? How would that change our lives? If for just one day you could wake up and look in that mirror and just feel happier about being you, how would that feel? I think that maybe relief and calm would be the result.

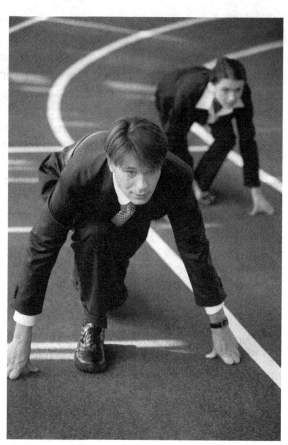

With this viewpoint we celebrate our uniqueness. We may look at others and admire them, respect them, and even try to emulate them. Part of the premise of neurolinguistic programming (NLP) is to look at people who have achieved the things you want in your life and to determine the habits that have enabled them to achieve that success. Then you model yourself on their habits. You do not try to become them. You take those qualities and make them your own. You cultivate your uniqueness and at the same time learn from others.

The Leaf's Journey

What is the leaf's purpose? It is to grow in its season, to feed the tree in its season, and to die in its season. It is a simple journey, one that fulfils its purpose, but one that serves another purpose too. For in living, the leaf serves the tree and the leaves that will follow it in years to come. It must bear the high winds, the lightning storms, and the chill of autumn to fulfil its purpose, but in so doing it enjoys the beautiful warmth of summer, the feeling of vitality of youth in spring, the surging power of water as it is drawn from the ground, and the vibrant colours of death before its final journey to the forest floor. It grows and owes its life to the leaves that went before it. It has a lineage, an ancestry to live up to. It knows none of this, but it feels it, and it lives its life in honour of the past and the future. Each leaf feeds the tree that gave it life. There is beauty in that, humility and love. Whatever adversity befalls it, the leaf still serves loyally, humbly, and with integrity. Only death can separate the leaf from the tree, and then it feeds the tree even then, a final gesture of love to the one that started it all.

We are leaves. We owe this great gift of life to our ancestors, and we have a debt of honour to pay to the generations of the future. Life will batter us, and life will love us, show us beauty and pain, give us all the nourishment we need, and give us purpose. What more can we ask? For in serving life, we feed the future, we honour the past, and we empower the present. We are witness to an incredible journey, our journey, and to a greater journey, one that we have the privilege to play a part in. Let us feed the one that gives us life, and let us honour that which honoured us with existence. Let us make it worthwhile. Let it mean something. Let it nourish, rather than poison. Let it grow, rather than diminish. Let us love, rather than hate.

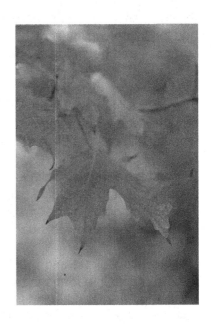

My Personal Journey

My personal journey with energy started with martial arts and Zen. As a teenager I was taught that there is a source to my creative power, and that it is my uniqueness, which is to be cultivated and nurtured throughout my life. As the years have passed, I have looked on in wonder at what I have been able to achieve in my life, thanks to the support from teachers and friends who continue to help me remove the shackles that have limited me in the past and in part still continue to limit me today. Slowly I remove them, freeing myself and allowing myself to become a fuller and more complete version of myself. Physical ability, performance ability, teaching ability, self-reliance, and self-belief have all been questioned by me and others. These things are with all of us. Sometimes I have been found lacking, and sometimes I have been able to bask in my strength and power. Life is full of both extremes.

To feel the full extent of our power, we must be free. The mind must not be tied to any concept; it must not be afraid to challenge and explore new ideas. In freeing ourselves, we open ourselves more fully to the experience of the moment. The more our energy is tied up in the concepts of the past, the more tired we become, the less present we become, and the less energy we have to express ourselves in this moment. This present moment is all there truly is. Fear of pain and fear of rejection are both powerful motivators that can come from the past; they can consume us and so deny us the wonder and enjoyment of the present.

These are the fears that I struggle with daily. When I am consumed by this fear, I feel the energy leave me. I have no strength for life and no excitement for it. For many years I have run from these fears, but I understand now that I do that out of fear of the pain I might feel. I may be overcome. I might even die!!!!! All I am doing is pushing me away from myself. I am denying what I feel, and in doing that I leave myself chained to the past that keeps influencing me, affecting me, driving me, motivating me, diminishing me, and keeping me away from my completeness. If I am to be all that I can be, I must be free. I must face those parts of myself that are in pain and so be whole once more.

For each one of us is born whole and complete and innocent. In our naivety we are drawn away from that fullness and that uniqueness, and we are taught the importance of conformity and fitting in, until we begin to lose our self. We are encouraged to look outward for confirmation, for acceptance, and for a sense of worth. We search and strive without success, because we are always using ever-changing external reference points, paths, and directions set by others. We use their standards, their desires, their values, and their principles, never our own. Only when we cease searching outside of ourselves and begin looking inward for our own answers do we use a more stable, consistent, and fulfilling internal compass and begin to set our own course based upon *our* values and beliefs.

Meditation, as well as martial arts and Zen, has helped me with that. With every day I grow stronger and more complete. Like a rising sun on the horizon, I am already whole, but I must pull myself up, fully face the world, and become aware and reconcile my completeness. At that point light will come to my world in all of its beauty and magnitude. I will be born spiritually at last.

What these three disciplines have given me is a connection to this power. a connection to the self as they call it in Zen. In Hinduism it is called "atman"; in the Kabbalah it is the point in the heart; the American Indians call it "medicine". There are countless names, but it is the same thing. I feel that instinctively we know this part of ourselves to be our true selves, and we protect it at all costs.

We are all weakest and most vulnerable when we are young, when injustices inflicted upon us are almost impossible for us to understand and to defend ourselves against. Feelings of abandonment, of not being heard, and of indifference wound us terribly and make us retreat behind defences that work well to protect this most precious part of ourselves. Yet the process of coming out from behind this protective wall later in life is hard. It is the process of becoming aware of the warmth and love that has been missing from our life for so long that enables us to do so.

Martial arts, Zen, and meditation have made me aware of this warmth, and many of the people along the way have shown me that the world is not a place to be afraid of. It takes time to truly trust, but the process is one of evolution, as I said earlier. It is a rising sun that seeks the world above the horizon to share its light and help to create life.

It is battle between the man-made part of me that tells me not to trust and the nature-made part of me that tells me to trust. I feel trust winning out. The force of this grows steadily day by day, glowing brighter and shedding more and more light on my world that has been in darkness for many years. This force is energy. Energy that comes from that is the source, the unified field. I feel myself connecting to it more often and in a more profound way. It is as if the sun shines brighter every day, allowing me to look with more clarity, letting me see more of the beauty, helping me witness more of the potential, and showing me what can be done. It will take a lifetime, so there is no easy and quick path. Often in life we do not really know if we are on the right path. What is important, I think, is that we know we are on a positive path and that we remain on a positive path, growing, developing, and cultivating ourselves until the end. That way we are open to all potential.

But what is this positive path? Life is not, and cannot be, a series of highs in a never ending spiral of elation. That is unrealistic and unsustainable. Life will not be a journey of successes without disappointments and failures. That belief is naive and impossible. Life is a mixture of all these things. We love, and our hearts are broken.

We try new things, and we succeed. However often we fail, we learn from our mistakes, and in turn we become more successful at those things that once eluded us. Apathy and indifference can often be the result of our failures, and we need to fight these things. This enables us to take pleasure and be pleased with our successes, and in turn we can discover something new and exciting about ourselves and about life along the way. Some days we are so high that we feel invincible, while other days we feel so low and feel worthless, as if life has been a complete waste of time. These dark days are not days to make important decisions or to act rashly and impulsively. Your thoughts are dark; do not act on them. To do so is to walk a negative path, and the consequences could be severe.

A great man told me once that pain is what you feel when you have lost someone or something that you love. Pain is not a negative thing. It shows your deep positive connection. Pain hurts, and sometimes it hurts so much that you would rather block it out. A lifetime of pain leaves you cold and isolated, for you cannot block out the pain without blocking out the love as well. We seek love and run from pain, yet we cannot have one without the other. This is the positive path—to feel the highs and lows of life. As a runner from pain all my life, I find this really hard, yet I know intuitively that it is right that we all have to have to experience pain sometimes.

I tell my students a wonderful story of a TV documentary about elephants. A female elephant has just given birth, and the herd must move quickly to a water hole three days' walk away, as they are in the middle of a drought and are in need of water. The baby valiantly walks, often in the shade offered by her mother between her legs. In the baking heat and with little milk from the mother because of her dehydrated state, the baby becomes weak and cannot walk any further. Resting in the shade of a tree, the baby finally dies. For four days the mother stands over the baby in what appears to be, to all intents and purposes, mourning. The rest of the herd waits for her at a respectful distance in spite of their need for water. Then suddenly the mother turns and walks away, and the herd rushes to the watering hole. It is a beautiful story of love and courage.

Pain is everywhere in nature, but nature does not give up. That mother elephant will have had another baby the following year, but at the same time she has been altered forever by the life and the death of her young cub.

In a culture of fear of pain, this is an almost impossible thing to imagine ourselves doing, and yet we do it. We have hope. We have a desire to touch and be touched. Whatever we might have done or experienced in the past that has left us disconnected, let us begin the process of reconnecting. It is hard, as if we are on the journey that Prince Charming has to make through the forest of brambles and thorns to reach Sleeping Beauty. Only by kissing her can we truly awaken the connection we have for life itself. I know I am in the forest, finding my way to the castle where she sleeps, and everything I do brings me a step closer to that moment. This is the positive path.

The knowledge in this book has strengthened my understanding about all of life. The meditations have strengthened my experience of the connection to the higher realms of energy and life. Zen peels away the falsehood of my mind, and martial arts allows me to feel the energy of my whole being soaring in movement.

Change Can Be Chaos

In-built change is present in the universe. All things change. You change. A tree changes. Everything changes. Nothing is truly static. Static and absolute stillness is an illusion. There is always change and movement throughout life, situations, and the Universe. This is important to understand, and we must always remember it. For in the best of your life or the worst of your life, no matter how long your life lasts or a situation lasts, things will indeed change one day. To understand this allows us to think and act in a manner that facilitates growth.

All of life and all situations do not repeat exactly the same. Physically, all life repeats slightly differently each time it changes. This enables deterioration or correction in all things. The clock starts ticking the moment any life form is born or created. It is born to deteriorate in form. It is also born to perfect, and it is born to grow through experience.

Experience is potential realised. The future is potential to be experienced. The present is the illusion of static experience. The future is undecided, waiting for you to take the energy in this direction or that. To feel the potential outcome of any situation or interaction, feel the energy of the situation or interaction. Use your own energy connection. Connect to the energy.

There is not death, just movement and experience from one form to another form of energy. You are energy.

Inner Voice and Energy Connection

For many years both my co-author and I have struggled individually with reconciling the demands that society would have us live by and the demands that listening to the inner voice urges us to fulfil. Rarely, if ever, do the two work in harmony, yet that is what we must all strive to achieve. We are brought up to live within the structure of conformity and fulfilling roles that other people think are best or most appropriate for us. Any individualism is quashed from an early age. It is deemed difficult, troublesome, different, or even unintelligent and pointless. These harsh judgements have a powerful effect on us, and our individual voice is silenced over time. We may go through life feeling unfulfilled and frustrated, as if life has no meaning, when deep down within us we feel that it does have meaning, as if it is a distant memory that is almost impossible to recall. We live in a society that powers up the voice that keeps this inner individualism silenced, and we listen to this voice as it is so loud and its message comes to us so frequently. We may even acknowledge the process ourselves.

The Inner Voice

This inner voice is alive and well inside you. I know it is, or you would not be reading this book. Reading this book implies you are searching for something! What are you searching for, do you think? It is a searching for that inner voice that is located deep inside of you. The purpose of the drive to do so is to help you discover your own true life's purpose. Once you have discovered your inner voice and have learnt how to trust it, it will help you discover that your life's meaning is something worthwhile, something meaningful to you. Throughout time, wise people have recognised this inner quality in both themselves and in others and have attempted to encourage this flame that requires constant attention and harnessing so that it becomes stronger and blazes bright in the world. You deserve to burn bright in the world, as that is the purpose of life for each of us. Mostly we are ordinary people who keep society ticking over for all. Whatever our role in society is, each of us has our place both within society and the wider Universe, and we each have our own unique purpose in life itself. The Chinese called it the Tao, the American Indians called it the Great Spirit, and the Aborigines called it the dreaming. Cultures across the world have countless names for it in their various tongues. In essence, it is a means to defining one's place in the world and how to find it.

Society offers us protection. It answers our needs on a very practical level, but in order to do so, it has to treat us all as the same or similar. It has to assume we want the same things, and we are encouraged to want the same things. None of this is wrong or bad; it is just that we are steered in a way that benefits society. Society demands obedience for its own survival, and we comply. But what about individual wants and individual paths? What about unique qualities, thoughts, and ideas? It is these that drive the world forward. It is the people who have them who find their place in the world and have the inner strength to speak out and make a difference. They are many, but they are not all of us.

We all have something to contribute, something to achieve, something to offer, something to be proud of that we can dedicate our lives to, and in so doing give our lives meaning. First we have to believe that this is so, and then we have to understand that there is a process to achieving the connection with our own life's path. You have already taken the first step, for you recognise that there is an inner voice within you that wishes to be heard. All you need to do is to listen to the voice inside of you, and a process begins. This process unfolds into a journey of wonderment and discovery. You are an incredible creature, and you are part of an incredible Universe. There is unlimited potential inside of you. Believing that this is so is the first step.

Your inner potential requires some work from you. It requires an uncovering of new depths, skills, and qualities that you may not realise you have. We all have this potential. We all have this ability to delve deep within ourselves and find out what we truly are. We all believe we are something (a son, a daughter, a mother, a father, a husband, a wife, a teacher, a plumber, an accountant, a window cleaner, a lawyer, a scientist, an artist), yet we may feel at a deep level that we are more. It takes time to uncover the truth. It takes a lifelong journey of learning, discovery, and wonder. We all need to uncover a kernel of truth that is the truth for all of us. It is a truth for all of creation.

A Kernel of Truth

There is a different way, one where each one of us can feel fulfilled and appreciated for the skills and qualities that we possess. To find this new way, we need to see ourselves differently. We need to grasp a different way of looking at the world. The way that I speak of here *is* reality. It is just not the way we are used to experiencing reality or even thinking about reality. What is required is a shift in thinking, even in perception.

This kernel of truth is that energy is the building block of the entire Universe. Energy underpins everything. Energy is the essence of the Universe. It is the one unifying, constituent ingredient of all things. Break all things down to their smallest parts, their base essence, and you are left with pure energy. It is fluid, dynamic, and powerful, and the key to our fulfilment is an understanding of this truth—not on an intellectual level, but on an experiential level. We can discuss theory, and we do so in this book, as it helps us to understand the argument. However, what the reality comes down to is practical skills. That means we learn to connect to this energy, work in harmony with this force of the Universe, and harness its power for our own betterment and the betterment of all.

Like Water

Working in harmony with this energy is a little bit like water in living organisms. Without water, living things cannot live. Water is the foundation of life on earth. Every cell that goes to make a tree, an insect, a cat, or a human must have sufficient water to work as it should and survive. Water comes out and water comes in in a highly regulated fashion. We breathe water out, we urinate, and we sweat, and we must replenish it by drinking water and other water-based fluids and by eating. We are an integrated part of the water system. We have it within us, and it flows and does its magic within us, but it also leaves and enters us by natural systems and actions. Imagine a fictitious situation where you are not playing your part in this system or cycle. The effect on the whole would be very small, almost unnoticeable, but that does not mean that we do not play our part. In fact, we have a role *because* we are here. The role is important because it is important that everything plays its part in the whole, but to mistakenly believe that we are all important is an illusion of the ego. In the grand scheme of things we are insignificant, but the very fact we are here means that it is important that we play our role as best we can. That is part of our purpose.

Isolation from the water system would be devastating. Without water coming in and water going out, the body would become poisoned and stagnated. With water only going out and no opportunity to replenish it, the body becomes weak and dehydrated and eventually stops functioning. If water only comes in, the person feels bloated and cannot release the stagnated and poisoned water within. If water cannot flow within you, it stagnates. There would be no free flow of blood and other fluids around the body, no chance of exchange of things in the water like nutrients, oxygen, or carbon dioxide, and in time the body would shut down and die.

Similar systems and actions exist in all living things and all around the planet. The currents of the oceans and the air shift massive volumes of water. Rivers and glaciers move water across land. Wind moves water in the air as moisture and cloud. Water evaporates from the surface of oceans, rivers, lakes, and the ground into the atmosphere. Plants draw water out of the ground and send it into the air. Rain, snow, hail, and other forms of precipitation send the water back to the earth's surface. This cycle is never-ending. The water within us has been recycled time and time again around the planet for millennia. We are part of the cycle of life.

Harnessing water is something nature has developed over time. It is the substance on which life is built. Through a process of development, nature has devised ways of using water and moving it around. If it does not move, it stagnates and becomes poisoned. Water is dynamic. It is gravity that makes it flow; it is our hearts and the winds that make it move; it is osmosis that makes it shift. These are the forces that drive water on this beautiful planet of ours.

Energy is not subject to the same restraints that water is under. It is not affected by gravity; it is gravity. It is not affected by wind; it is the wind. It is without mass, it is without form, and yet it is the building block of all matter and form in the universe.

Energy moves using its own systems and actions, but the idea of moving water is not dissimilar to moving energy. It flows in and out and within all things. It is between all things. It means that things can interact through this flow of energy. Music that excites you makes you feel more energised. Colours that calm you make you feel more serene. A room with a wood theme feels very different to a room with metal furniture.

This is the realm of this book. By seeing the world from an energy perspective, we can see how all things are interrelated and intertwined. Nothing is isolated. All things are connected. We live in a beautiful network of systems that are working in relation to each other in harmony. We can become aware of something greater and can become aware that we are part of something greater than perhaps we at first realised.

Recall the idea of water not flowing freely within you, into you, and out of you. If we exchange the idea of water with energy, we have a similar scenario. The only difference is that the lack of energy movement does not kill us, but it does diminish our power and strength and so limits our potential. Again, it is important to stress that we play our part in this system and that we play it to the best of our ability. We have a responsibility to ourselves and to others to share in the energy around us and to fuel it as positively as we can. To opt out of this is not to fulfil our role in the grand scheme of things. "What can I do?" I hear you ask. Well, that is part of each individual's journey. By understanding the many subtle and not-so-subtle ways in which energy works is to gain an appreciation of the tasks awaiting you in life and how to go about them, how to live a life with integrity, honour, compassion, and trust.

Quality of Energy

Think of yourself as a rechargeable battery. Batteries work best and last longer if you drain them and replenish them. To do this the energy flows through it, as well as into it and out of it. The energy levels of the body need recharging and must be used up too. We recharge with food and sleep. Good quality sleep revitalises the body, just as good nutrient rich food fuels the body. Exercise and daily living use up this energy and drain the charge from the battery, but it is this daily living that gives us our excitement and passion for our life, which is another form or quality of energy altogether. Our passion for life must be fuelled too. We must be fed from the activities in our lives, from life itself, from the people we are with, and from the places we go to, and part of the cycle is that we feed them. We find power sources for this energy in our nurturing and loving relationships, in our positive working relationships and roles, in our hobbies for which we have passion, and, if we are lucky, in the jobs for which we have passion. We can be drained by all forms of negative relationships, by jobs that make us feel undervalued, and by environments that do not support and nurture us. The energy flows out as well as in.

Just as water has different qualities, so does energy. Relationships at work and at home can be supportive or not. They can undermine and bolster and invigorate. It depends on the quality of the relationship. We know whether a relationship with someone is doing us good or not. A positive relationship makes us feel great. Though we may argue and disagree, there is mutual support, respect, and love for the other person. In a negative relationship, there is only undermining, blame, and chastising. The energy and the quality of the relationships are fundamentally different. They feed us differently, and make us feel different. They fuel the battery with a certain quality of energy, and that energy is the energy that will come from the battery. In short, what goes in must come out.

To feel empowered in a work or personal relationship feels fantastic. To feel great about yourself feels wonderful. This is the effect energy has on us, not just physically but also emotionally.

Sensing Energy

To begin with, we must become aware of energy itself. We are surrounded by it, and our senses are adapted to interpret this energy into sight, sound, taste, touch, and smell. Sight is simply the retina in the eye receiving light (electromagnetic energy) information, which is sent to a certain part of the brain through the optic nerve, which then interprets those signals as a picture. Sound waves (carrying energy) move through the air and touch the ear drum, sending signals via the auditory nerve to the brain, which interprets these sounds as language, music, laughter, a bird singing, and so on. Our senses are highly adapted to generating a certain picture of the world around us, and our brains are highly skilled at interpreting this information based upon our perception and understanding of the world.

As science will tell us, there is a whole range of areas on the electromagnetic spectrum that are invisible to us, as there are sounds that we cannot hear. We do not perceive them, but it does not mean they are not there, and it does not mean that they do not affect us and influence us in ways that we do not understand. Just as water enters us, so too does energy. Energy does not follow the rules water must follow. Energy does not have to enter the body through the mouth and come out through the pores of the skin. It can enter anywhere, and it can leave anywhere. This process is happening all the time. Even as I write this, the electromagnetic waves from the computer are radiating from it and entering me. Whatever energy is within me is radiating out into the room—my thoughts, my feelings, and my emotions. The sounds in the building and the sounds and light from outside all contribute to the flow of energy that is the flow of life and being in the universe.

If we think of people emitting energy, think of that energy as a colour. Waves of energy are coming out of us all the time. The colour changes as we change. There are subtle changes in shade and hue as we go about our days and our lives. These waves enter a vast sea of energy that in a close environment is relatively concentrated. As it expands out, it becomes more and more diluted until it "seems" there is none there. There is though. That is the point. Each wave contributes to the whole. What do you want to contribute? What colour do you want the Universe to be? Your thoughts and feelings, emotions, and mental states all affect the colour of the energy within you, and so they affect the colour that emanates from you into the sea of being.

The Power of Thought

What affects the colour within you? What affects the energy within you? Your thoughts are exceptionally powerful. As you create them, they generate waves that radiate into the world. All your thoughts are doing this all of the time, not just your daily surface-level thoughts, but also the deeper-seated beliefs and values that drive you and your behaviour. Negative-thinking people seem to exude negativity. Positive-thinking people feel positive and attract positive people. Self-limiting beliefs limit us because we believe them to be true, and so we act upon that supposed truth. These thoughts pervade us and so dominate or underpin how we think, feel, and behave not just to ourselves, but also to others. The quality of energy that we have affects others. Our energy level and the quality of the energy within us are affected by the way we think and feel.

Translate this into a colour, and that would be the colour within you and the colour you put out into the world. Some people refer to this colour as the aura. The aura is simply energy. It is in fact, electromagnetic energy. Some people pick it up through feel, while others "see" it as colour in a field around things. You may feel this energy in a wooded glade, in a nightclub when a fight is about to start, perhaps in a church, mosque, synagogue, or temple, at a pop concert or a sporting event, or even in a gentleman's club or a roadside café. If you "see" it, then you already know what I am talking about! Our internal environment is very important. Therefore, management of our thoughts and feelings is very important, and the meditations in this book will help you to manage your state of mind and thus your internal environment. Our internal environment becomes translated to the energy that others either see or feel on the outside of us by way of our auras.

Awareness of Energy

Your body needs to be fit and healthy, powerful, and supple. Regular exercise and eating a balanced nutritious diet are essential for the body's vitality. People who exercise regularly are usually more energetic. They have a better positive outlook and are generally more productive. A healthy diet can help to bolster the immune system, aids recovery better from injury or illness, facilitates better sleep, and provides more energy during the day. Our external environment is just as significant—our friends and family, our home and work environments, the clothes we wear, the places we visit, and the things we do. All of these affect our energy, because the energy of these things affects the energy of our bodies. Some of the meditations in this book highlight health, and as we become more sensitive to the flowing energy around us, we learn to become more in tune with the energy of the things around us and within us. Awareness is the key, and the meditations in this book will help to awaken and develop your awareness of the energy around you.

Once you are aware, then you will begin to realise and understand how energy moves and flows and how you can play your part in that. You cannot dominate energy through force of will. You have to understand the ways in which it flows and how you can move it around consciously, with the goal of moving through the world in peace and harmony, in humility and compassion.

We do not claim to have a definitive answer and explanation for all the ways in which energy works and its manifestations. Purely on a physical level, all things are made up of atoms, which are themselves made up of energy. Atoms vibrate, and they gain the endless fuel for this by absorbing heat from the environment around them. Somehow, larger objects have developed a structured energy system within them, such as the chakra system explained in Chinese and other oriental cultures. We have no idea how these systems have come into being, but evidence suggests that they do exist and that we ignore them at a great cost to our health and our well-being. Built around these cultures are practises that increase the power of the energy and the flow of that energy within people. Yoga, Reiki, martial arts, chi Kung, and meditation itself are all energy-enhancing practises that have been developed in the East. Historically, Western medicine and psychology have under-estimated the power of energy, but they are now beginning to acknowledge the diverse ways in which it can be used for people's physical, mental, and emotional health. Eastern medicine's goal is to keep the energy flowing, for this is the recipe for a healthy and balanced living organism. The planets, solar systems, galaxies, and the universe as a whole are subject to the same requirements.

The alternative to flowing energy is stagnation. It either flows or it does not. Just as water spoils when it stagnates, so too does energy. It stagnates in the muscles and minds of people in the form or stress, tension, and ill health. In no other place in nature does this stagnation take place that we know of. It is a product of humanity. We have much to learn from nature. We need to rest and play, as well as work.

120

We must do all three when it is time. Get the balance of all three points. The triangle moves constantly, moving the water all the time. There is no chance for stagnation, only an ever-increasing triangle of power that keeps us in harmony. Too much of anything makes us imbalanced. Too much work is a common fact of life for many people these days. This encourages the water to stagnate in one corner. In this instant world of "must have it now", there is often not enough rest, or among the long-term unemployed, there is too much inactivity. In an environment of deadlines and targets, there is not enough time to play or to be with family and friends. All three must remain in balance, or else the energy stagnates.

And we must connect. You perhaps now understand that all of the meditations connect us to ourselves, to our environment, to our greater self, and to the greater Universe. With connection comes communication, and with communication comes an exchange of energy that we can become aware of at a conscious level. The more deeply we connect, the more profound our communication. Indeed, we experience something spiritual in our everyday living. The meditations in this book have taken you on this journey. They have taken you deeper and deeper into the truth of the universe, and energy is the core of that truth. Energy is the platform on which the universe is built. All things are supported by energy. Without energy there would be nothing ("no thing"). We, the human race, are the furthest that energy has managed to explore, the most powerful thing that energy has been able to support. What makes us so special? We have conscious thought, and we know it. We have awareness that is, as far as we know, a unique attribute of any creature on the planet. And, just like everything else, awareness and conscious thought are both supported by energy. They *are* energy. So they must follow the rules that energy must follow. The rules are as follows.

1. Energy flows.

Energy follows paths that are created by conditions. Galaxies, stars, and planets are created through the timely coordination of conditions. All the right bits need to be in the right place, and—bang!—we have a galaxy forming, a star, a planet, an atom, or life itself. Conditions allow the energy to flow in a given direction, and that is what creates creation. Think of an electrical appliance. Once it is made, once the conditions are right, the energy flows through it and it works. In other words, connect it to the electricity and the appliance starts to work as conditions allow. Life is the same. Conditions are right for life or they are not. The energy flows to sustain life, and if conditions are not right, the energy flows differently and life cannot be sustained. This is the brutal truth of nature, and there is a beauty in the simplicity of it, especially for those of us blessed with the gift of life and aware enough to want to explore this wonderful gift we have been given.

2. Flowing energy creates waves, just as a boat cutting through the water will create waves that radiate out and interact with other waves. Light and sound are classic examples of energy travelling through space in waves. Different qualities of sound and light waves will have different wavelengths.

Energy Flow

Awareness and conscious thought are tools that can manipulate energy. They can be used to create conditions through which energy will flow. Energy requires sustained thought and awareness, not just a blip. Think of how long it took to create our beautiful planet earth or the sun. It required sustained "thought" or, rather, sustained conditions that allowed the energy to take form in the way that it has. As conditions have subtly changed, so the energy has flowed subtly differently, and so the earth and the sun have evolved into the things that they are today.

Your life works the same way. Your conscious mind has the ability to think in a sustained direction. The thoughts that you have will take time to create, and they can be created because you will think of them over a period of time; you will break down a goal into smaller parts to be able to achieve the greater goal.

Man has an incredible ability to create poetry and literature, space ships and cars, buildings like the Empire State or the Taj Mahal, wisdom and beauty like that of Gandhi or Buddha, as well as the horrors of Adolf Hitler or Slobodan Milosovic. This ability is our human gift and our human curse, and not just in action. For our thoughts send ripples out that affect others and interact with others in far more subtle ways than actions do.

Take for example a concert. The atmosphere at an opera or an orchestral recital is very different to that of a rock concert. Why? Even before the performance has started, the anticipation in the audience is very powerful, as hundreds or even thousands of people think about what is going to happen. This affects the crowd, which in turn affects the performers. When the performers play, they affect the crowd still more, and so the ambience spirals into a mutually enhancing experience. This is the power of the energy of the mind, as well as the music. Why do you think so many performers have warm-up acts? Comedians want the crowd to be in a receptive mood before they step on the stage. The warm-up act does that, or at least that is what he is paid for, so that the audience is focussed in a light-hearted and humorous atmosphere for the main act. All this is the movement and manipulation of energy. In entertainment it is an art form.

Perhaps that is why crowds develop a group mentality. Sporting events are very similar. When hooligans incite a crowd to violence, it is their thoughts of violence that infect others, and soon the ambience of excitement and enthusiasm is replaced with one of anger and aggression. Hitler, Idi Amin, and Milosovic took it to a national or even an international level, but the principle is the same. Gandhi, Martin Luther King, and Aung San Suu Ki affected crowds and nations in a nonviolent manner.

It is the power of thought, and thought is energy. Energy feeds minds, builds nations, and creates planets and solar systems. It creates life, of which death is a natural part, and it creates lives, futures, relationships, and passion. That is its power. Once we learn to harness it, we can unleash the potential that lies within all of us. This is a worthy quest, a necessary journey, and the opportunity to discover what truly lies within.

There is a vitality, a life force, an energy, a quickening, that is translated through you into action, and because there is only one of you in all time, this expression is unique.

—Martha Graham

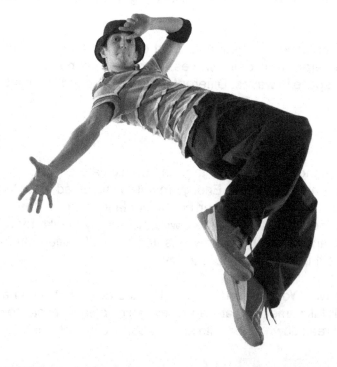

Where Is the Magic?

"Inexplicable or remarkable influence producing surprising results"—that is the dictionary definition of magic. A bit boring, I must say. For if we just say the word "magic" in our minds, it conjurers up beauty and wonder. It is exciting and wondrous. It conjures up tinsel and sparkle, the like of which is too much to behold. Christmas is magical; the theatre is magical; our birthdays are magical, as are all celebrations in general. Passing our driving test is magical. Passing an exam for which we have worked hard is magical. Falling in love is magical. Giving birth or becoming a parent is magical. Strolling in the park on a summer's day is magical—or even on a cold winter's day with a bite in the air. Smelling a sweet-scented rose is magical. Spending time with dear friends can be magical. Watching your child's first steps can also be magical. What could you add to this list? Add them now. For each of us there are many magical things in life. We encounter many things that can make our days wonderful. The things that make our time on earth wondrous are most often not material at all. They are achievements and connections with others or with the earth.

As an artist, I have been taught to look at the world. I do not mean look, or just look, but *really* look. How many of us do this? Not many, I think. Maybe I am wrong, but I do not see people really looking. A good friend of mine who is a research scientist told me about the beauty that she sees down the lens of a microscope. My friend said that the average person does not get to see what she sees and has seen. She said that there is a beauty down the microscope lens equal to any the rest of us could see, should we care to look, out in the wider world.

I have always appreciated the world around me for as long as I can remember. The form of flowers, the shape of bugs, and the colour of birds has set my heart racing more often than not. A shiny new car is a thing to covet, but its beauty for me is not a patch on the earth's own products. How often is the natural beauty of the earth blindly unobserved by so many of us? When an artist or designer looks for inspiration, it is in the natural world that they look more often than not. To learn their trade, they are encouraged and sometimes forced to look, look, look around them at the natural beauty of the world. The more one looks deeply, the more one sees of the wonder of the earth. The simplest things encountered can bring the greatest joy in any person's heart. As I sit here writing this, there is a fly that has landed on my desk. It is in the process of dying. Its body is upturned, and he is fighting to turn over. This is life in action. He has served his purpose, and now he has landed on my desk and is sharing his end with me. He is just a little fly, and most of us would normally reach for the fly swatter and give him a good and swift end, but not today. Today I will observe the beauty of his last moments and allow him to have them in peace. Life has many moments, all of varying qualities. Some have magic and beauty, others quiet and calm, and others turbulence and disturbance. All of those moments play their part. All of the moments that you have at your disposal are yours to use as you wish. They are there for you to observe magic or close your eyes to it. The magic will always be around you just waiting for you to open your eyes and enjoy. When you are indeed ready, the magic is there to share itself with you. Above all of this wondrous magic that is around you waiting to share itself with you is you. For you are magical also. You are part of this wondrous magic. *How magical is that?*

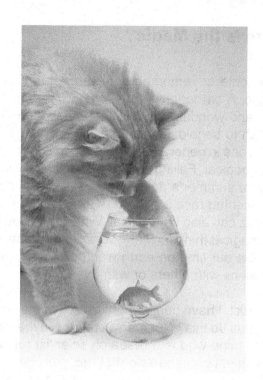

> *We weren't put here to be miserable. We were put here to do the best we can, and we should take our energy and improve our state of being.*
>
> —Lenny Kravitz

Stagnating Energy

Man, in his obsession with identity, restricts the flow of energy, and this is poisonous to him. This often results in ill health, and ill health is a great problem for man. Identity means ownership, and man cannot own what was here before he was, and neither can he own what will remain after he has gone. This was the American Indian, Aborigine, and Maori argument about land when the white man came. The white man asked who owned the land, and the indigenous populations said that no one owns the land, so the white man took the land. He then threw the indigenous peoples off their ancestral homes and killed them when they fought to protect the balance that had sustained them for millennia.

Identity leads to ownership and possession. In his life, a person has to move from dependence through independence and mature into interdependence. The last is the greatest level of man, the level that nature understands intuitively. We can achieve far more together than we can alone. Independence is essential for interdependence and comes from an inner strength, the self-knowledge and belief that allow us to surrender our fear-driven needs for a greater idea. Dependency (emotional, financial, and physical) is the state of children, but so many of us do not grow beyond this stage in adulthood, particularly emotionally. This motivates fear in us, for we think we cannot survive without this other person. How wrong we are! But we must grow to become independent and evolve to become interdependent.

Trying to live by that which society says is the most acceptable way of living encourages people to be dependent. People often become dissatisfied with themselves as they try to measure up in one way or another to society's benchmarks—the best job, the best clothes, the best physical look, being able to afford plenty of it all, never being allowed to just be satisfied with what they have and always being encouraged to strive for something else. This can be seen as negative energy flow, as continual dissatisfaction causes stress, and stress in the end will cause stagnation, as there is never peace and harmony within the person.

In stagnation, man poisons his soul, his body and his mind. The poison spreads to infect the planet. Like stagnant water, the energy begins to spoil, and it manifests in the body as tightness in muscles, sustained levels of stress within the body, a suppressed immune response, and an increase in the incidence of illness and disease. In the mind it manifests as irritability, inappropriate anger, and violence, a disregard for others and oneself. When we disconnect spiritually, we think and feel ourselves to be separate, and so we act in destructive and harmful ways. So what flows from stagnation is negative energy, just as stagnant water carries the poison within it when it begins to flow again.

To combat stagnant energy flow, we need to strive to fight negative energy by encouraging others and ourselves to maintain a positive attitude. We must control the flow of negativity, limiting it as best we can. By working on ourselves positively, we open the way to the flow of positivity, and as we come into balance as a result, in turn we act according to balance. To enable us to achieve the desired balance, we must fight our inclination to resist change and our indifference towards the effort required to create change. Apathy is a massive force in the world today. We must fight it, for it leads to stagnation of energy and further negativity. Indigenous people knew that one needs to keep things in balance and harmony. Then the energy flows correctly both in man and within the environment. *We must bother. We must care.*

Philanthropic

The best thing that anyone can do in creating their own life is to be philanthropic. For those people out there in life who do not know the meaning of that word, and there are lots of you, the dictionary definition is; loving ones fellow men benevolent, humane. Please write it on a piece of paper and sit with it in your hands. Peruse this meaning. Ask yourself what it means. You are it sometimes, and yet if I ask you to give a definition of this word and explain it to me not using the dictionary definition but your own definition drawn from your own experience, you would indeed find it hard. I would find it hard. What does it mean to be humane? What does it mean to love one's fellow man?

It means to put others first before yourself. It means to not have a selfish outlook on life. It means to have a piece of bread and to cut it into three and share it three ways with two others—not just half with one other person. This is not an easy thing to do, for there is the survival mechanism with which we are all programmed. This tells us to be for ourselves, for being so gives us the greatest chance of survival. We turn against our own in the bid to be the one to survive this life. We are told that there are plenty of resources on the earth to feed us all but that, with the increase in the world's population, the earth maybe will not be able to sustain that growth in the future. It is a scary prospect that the world's resources are dwindling and will become even shorter as time goes on. Surely then we will all become more selfish as we each will store up for ourselves that which we need to survive. Our own survival is paramount, and that of our neighbour is not our concern. Surely this is so?

Who would volunteer to live in this life alone? To be without empathy is to be without humanity. To be without love is to be without human connection. To live a selfish life, one has to cultivate these qualities. One has to be prepared to cut off oneself off from the pain that one inflicts on one's fellow man. We must be prepared to inflict pain and walk away and revel in our own spoils. We must be prepared to sit in our own dark cupboard by ourselves and laugh with glee at the spoils which we have gathered for ourselves by using any means. We must then fatten ourselves and clothe ourselves with the spoils which have made us rich. We must turn our backs on our good work and walk on by, while the evidence of our actions sits in the gutter as we walk past.

I have no answer for you as to how we should apportion our wealth and food. I am no wiser than you. I just know that we are each selfish and cruel. I have lived a fairly long time and have seen many things and met many people along the way. The selfishness of people never ceases to amaze me. It never ceases to shock me when the hand of friendship is bitten off time and time again. We are indeed each in our own space within life. We all have our own position in society and in life itself. However, the thing that binds us together is our humanity. It is the golden thread that binds us to our neighbour. If we sever that thread, what are we left with? We are left with emptiness, disillusionment, and abandonment. We are left with a void that will never be filled by any amount of beautiful objects. Beauty is in the eye of the beholder, it has been said. But to exchange one beauty for another does not necessarily balance the scales.

Before we lose our personal or collective dignity or even our humanity itself, we all need to think long and hard about what it means to be human. What does it mean to us personally or globally or nationally? I had a conversation with my chi Kung teacher about a story in the news recently that reported boys as young as eight cage fighting. Oh my goodness, what are we all becoming? Are we all turning into hard-hearted brutal monsters? Are we now people of no humanity? Have we become people of no conscience? Life is tough, but not so tough that we have to brutalise and teach our children to be brutal people.

There are so many children across the planet who never know what childhood is. They look after families by enslaving themselves or being enslaved to a life of hardship and servitude. They are brutalised, neglected, and forgotten. They are exploited beyond endurance. Each of us in the West has some part in this misery. Children and people are not property to be exploited. I have no answer to this sad state of affairs. It is one that humanity has organised for itself and brought upon itself. It is all of our own doing, and that is the truth. For if it is not our fault, then who are we to blame? Maybe we can each blame the other person? Why not? It is easy to do that.

We create our own lives each day. Action upon action builds a life. Our thoughts and our feelings create us. That collectively creates life on Planet Earth. There have been many good people in history that have walked a good path. Those people have tried so hard to share something of the goodness that resided deep within them. They tried to show each of us something special about ourselves. To find these people, look to your religious or history books. There are so many of them. Need and greed and want seem to blind us to their fundamentally true message—that we must coexist here on this earth for this time and that we must try to do so with grace, dignity, harmony, and love for all in our hearts.

At the heart of this is the word "respect"—respect for ourselves, respect for the privilege of being a human being, and respect the ability to give and to share. I promise you, money comes and money goes. *C'est la vie.* That's for sure.

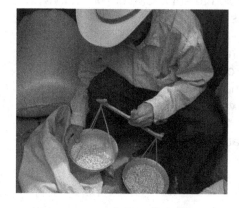

All virtue is summed up in dealing justly.

—Aristotle

Energy is Everywhere

The universe came from nothing, emptiness, a void. Any physical object is simply a vibration of that void; its essence is emptiness. The only thing that gives it substance is vibration. The thing you feel when you meet someone or read something or look at a picture or a landscape is the vibration that created it, which is, at its essence, void. All that you are is the sum of your vibration at this moment. The thoughts you are having that either draw you further and further from the moment or bring you closer and closer to its presence are vibration. To be completely present is to feel the powerful surge of energy that is the moment. It will knock your socks off. There is no room for anything else. There is no mortgage, no financial issues, and no worry about children, work, the leaking roof, or the blocked drain. Your entire being is absorbed in the now. This is our true state. This is our true power and our true potential. Whatever we choose to do, when we are in this state we will do it with our whole being.

Most often we are scattered. Our thoughts are on many things, when, in fact, to get anything done effectively, we need to focus on that one thing completely. When it is done, move on to the next and give it our full attention, our whole heart, and our entire being.

Learning to connect to our soul through meditation will allow this process to occur. In time we step into our self and realise our fullest potential. It takes time dedication, patience, and compassion, for we have a lifetime of understanding how to live.

The way we think influences the flow of energy. Meditation consciously draws the energy in, holds it, moves it, concentrates it, and lets it energise the body. These are neutral thoughts that will allow the energy to empower us. Whether they are positive or negative is up to us. Controlling what you think is vitally important. Negative reactions damage us, our bodies, our lives, and those around us who share our lives. Instead, mental, conscious control of the mind will lead to an empowered positive reaction that improves our health, our energy, our healing, our lives, and the lives of others' in general.

Energy does not care, as it is incapable of caring. It Is. It will flow wherever it can flow and will be used for whatever it can be used for. That is how the universe has been created and how it has evolved. It is incredible to think what can be created when infinite potential is on hand. From a lifeless universe came life. From a universe without consciousness came consciousness. That is the power of potential, and that potential is a manifestation of that universal energy.

The Way, the Dao, Being, the Great Spirit, God, the Dreaming—it has many names. It builds on an ever-lengthening spiral called *time*. It builds on one generation to build the next. No moment is ever the same.

This is what we are born into but never leave. We are witness to it. Enjoy it, for you will never witness it again. *The universe will move on, and so too will you.*

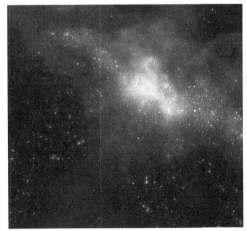

Just as there is no loss of basic energy in the Universe, so no thought or action is without its effects, present or ultimate, seen or unseen, felt or unfelt. —Norman Cousins

Set 4: Meditations for Self-Awareness

Self-Awareness Meditations Explained

These meditations are all about you. They are about being aware of who you are and your true potential.

The first meditation gives you your unique voice. It helps you to find your own voice that is deep inside of yourself. To be able to speak up for yourself and speak your own mind and truth, you have to have confidence in your own worth and validity. This is not easy. Many people are cut off from their own voice at childhood. Some of us are encouraged to say what we think and are encouraged to be part of the world and have a valid place in it. Others are positively discouraged from this. "Children should be seen and not heard." "Be quiet and speak when you are spoken to." "Shut up! Who do you think you are?" These sorts of teachings do not encourage us to be ourselves and speak for ourselves. Many adults have to learn how to speak up for themselves and find their own inner confidence. This meditation will help to facilitate that.

The second meditation helps you find your unique self. It is there and it is part of you. Finding it and, more importantly, expressing it are very hard to do for many people. We are told so often that only some chosen people are unique and have valid gifts. This is not true. You are unique, and you too have gifts. You just need to believe you are unique and have gifts, and you must dig deep and find them. Take the time to do this meditation, and it will help you see who you truly are.

The third meditation will help you to facilitate calmness. For life to treat us calmly, we must treat it so. Life offers so many challenges that challenge our calm and centeredness. This meditation will help to restore your sense of calm and balance when life helps to toss them out of the window.

Meditation 1: Accessing the Inner Voice

It is not easy to access your inner voice, your own inner strength. This meditation is to help you find your own true voice.

1. Take yourself down into relaxation.

2. Breathe slowly and deeply.

3. Start counting your breaths.

4. Focus on your inhalation and your exhalation.

5. Clear your mind of thoughts and worries.

6. Take yourself down as far as you can go.

7. Connect to your essence.

8. Focus on your solar plexus.

9. Build your energy centre. Fill it with white light energy and allow the energy to spread throughout your body. Allow the energy to gently energise your body.

10. Imagine your body growing and becoming larger. Allow your body to take all of the room it needs in the world.

11. Focus once again on your breath.

12. Breathe slowly and deeply.

13. Fill your chest.

14. Breathe out slowly.

15. Once again focus on the solar plexus.

16. Grow the energy and send it throughout your body.

17. Allow the energy to travel slowly, and let it once again energise you.

18. Now imagine you are a tall tree or building.

19. Take your own space.

20. Take your place in the world. Grow your roots, and lay down your foundations.

21. Anchor yourself to the ground.

22. Now once again breathe slowly, and deeply count the breaths.

23. Now that you are anchored and strong, take up nourishment and nutrients into your body from the earth below. Allow these nutrients to nourish your mind and your body. This will make you strong. To grow we need nourishment, and we draw this up from below.

24. Now concentrate on your breath. Again breathe slowly and deeply. Count the breaths.

25. .Now see the tree growing it gains its leaves. The leaves are a direct product of the nutrients you have drawn up from the earth below.

26. To grow strong, feel the mind and feel the body. You have all that you need. You are all that you need.

27. Take yourself down further into relaxation. Picture yourself as a strong person. Picture yourself in control of all that you do—all that you say, all that you think, all that you are.

28. Know that you are one of many. Know that you are one. Know that you are unique. Know that you have a right to be yourself.

29. Now gently and slowly allow yourself to come back to the here and now.

Meditation 2: The Unique Self

1. Take yourself down into relaxation.

2. Slowly count your breaths.

3. Breathe slowly and count the breaths as you breathe.

4. Allow the breath to gently and slowly take you down into an altered state of awareness.

5. Expand your aura to reach out to others. Feel the beauty of all that there is. This is part of you; this is not all of you. You are a unique individual.

6. Once again breathe deeply.

7. Allow the air to sit in the lungs for a moment before expulsion.

8. Slowly let the air out.

9. Take your mind back to past memories.
   Find one that pleases you and that makes you happy. Find a memory that connects you to yourself when you felt at home in your own skin. This memory of yourself shows your individuality. It shows you as the purest part of yourself. This is who you are and this is
   who you have a right to be.
   Know you have your own inner light.
   Know you have your own inner beauty.
   Know you have a right to be yourself.

10. Take some deep breaths in and out, and slowly let your breath out.

11. Breathe in and breathe out.

12. Stay in this state of relaxation for a while.

13. Reflect on your individual beauty. Understand you bring something good to the world. You bring yourself. This is who and what

14. you need to give. No more and no less.Ponder these thoughts and write them on your soul. Commit them to memory.Wake up when you feel it is right for you to do so. Wiggle your toes, feel your body, and come back to the here and now.

Meditation 3: The Calm Self

1. Take yourself down into relaxation.

1. Count your breaths.

2. Keep your eyes open and find a point of focus as you find your inner point of relaxation.

3. Breathe slowly and deeply to relax your body.

4. Fix your gaze on an object of beauty—a tree, a scene, a picture, an ornament.

5. Now slowly move your eyes to examine the beauty. Do not think as you do this. Allow no thoughts to enter your head. Just allow your eyes to absorb the beauty of the object of attention.

6. Now once again breathe slowly and deeply.

7. Now fix your gaze so that it is static and on one point of focus.

8. Allow the eyes to relax and go out of focus.

9. Breathe slowly and surely.

10. Be in this quiet space for as long as you feel the need to be.

Come back to the here and now when you feel ready to do so.

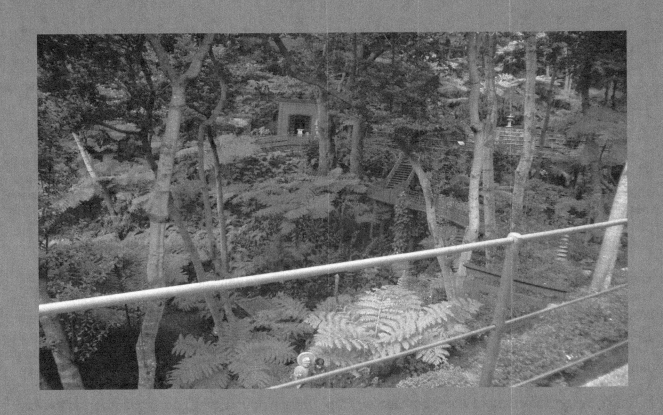

The true warrior learns how to correctly perceive the activity of the Universe and how to transform martial techniques into vehicles of purity, goodness and beauty. A warrior's mind and body must be permeated with enlightened wisdom and deep calm.

—Morihei Ueshiba

The Power

The Japanese understood the power of the Way. It is the method by which a man can access and power the self. Highly ritualised, it demands accurate proficiency, overcoming all boundaries of the ego, and entering into the world of the void, in which dwell consciousness and being. The word "do" in Japanese means "the Way". Aikido, judo, and karate-do are examples of Japanese martial arts in which a student could learn to become one with his opponent and himself, and in so doing transcend self and become one with all things. It demanded adherence to principles that brought a man to greatness.

This wisdom is not the reserved privilege of martial artists. That is why the Japanese "do" is so diverse. The tea ceremony (sado), archery (kyudo), calligraphy (shodo), and flower arranging (kado) are all practised, often in conjunction with martial arts, as to the Japanese there is no distinction between them. The martial arts cultivate spirit in the realm of violence, while the other arts cultivate spirit in peace and harmony. The Japanese understood that they are two sides of the same coin, and in the world of feudal Japan, it was essential for a man to be in harmony during times of war as well as in times of peace.

In China, the equivalent word would be "Dao" or "Tao". Taoism, founded by Lao Tzu, embodied the idea of Tao, the Way or the Path, and from that, martial arts like kung fu were born, as were principles in Chinese medicine such as acupuncture, acupressure, feng shui, and herbal medicine. The use of qi, or chi, is fundamental to these disciplines. Breathing is used as a method for improving the flow of chi energy through the body, as is attention to physical technique. This is also true of the Japanese Way, and "kiai" is the breathing used in Japanese martial arts styles, the kanji characters relating to harmony or union of spirit.

Whichever culture you adopt, whichever discipline you might follow (and there are many more than the ones cited here), the chosen way or path demands investment in oneself. To be truly great, one has to advance beyond self. Ego and self are invested in the past and future. Only the present can truly unleash the power of being. The ritual of the chosen way is designed to bring the student into the present and in so doing, it allows him to feel his true power and the power of the moment around him. The purpose is to learn and perfect for the sake of learning and perfection, not for prizes, trophies, or prestige, but rather for dominion over self, to be greater than oneself.

> To be great without glory
> To be powerful without position
> To "Be", without reward, in fact, to "Be" is reward enough.

It meant the student accessed the true source of all things. It was pure and therefore more powerful for it. What man could fight the Way? No man of the Way would need to fight, just to "be" is enough.

Wikipedia divides art into two categories, the motivated (art created for a practical purpose or reason) and the non-motivated (art created as part of the expression of being human). Motivated art can be seen as a means of communication, for entertainment, for psychological or healing purposes, or for the practical need to defend oneself, one's family and friends, or one's ideas and principles. For many people, martial arts' sole purpose is for the defence of one's personal safety. They focus on the "martial" side of martial arts, and this is indeed a purpose and may well have been the motivating force behind many styles. However, I have been taught that there is a deeper purpose behind martial arts, one that touches on the non-motivated criteria of art as well. Learning forms, principles, ideas, concepts, strategies, tactics, and techniques until they become a part of you is the "martial" side, and in time and with direction it leads to something deeper—the "art" of martial arts, by which a student can explore

- The basic human instinct for harmony, balance, and rhythm

- Experience of the mysterious

- Expression of the imagination

- Universal communication

- Ritualistic and symbolic functions

These are all central concepts to many forms by which an artist of whatever discipline practises the practical aspects of his or her art—the practicalities of oils and watercolours, different painting and drawing styles, uses of rhythm in music and poetry, the nuance of different instruments and tools, differing dance genres, etc.—until the artist finds within it the window for self-expression, that unique quality that makes your art your own, something different, something unique. You become at one with the techniques that you spent a lifetime honing, and doing so places you in "the zone" or the "flow" of no thought, no tension, no worry, no future and no past, but simply the moment, a connection with something universal, the experience of the mysterious, for it is beyond definition and need only be felt to be understood.

To practise these arts for glory, fame, or fortune is to diminish what is truly beautiful about them. It is the feeling of abandon that is the true motivator, the release from our petty worries and concerns, the chance to express something that is true to our nature and therefore profound. These are acts beyond ego. It is in the expression of art for art's sake that the truly great works are created. Fame and fortune come as a consequence of one's passion and one's love of the process, not as the result. We become lost in the process, and we enjoy the sensation of that process. The feeling of a brush stroke, a dance move, or a punch or kick becomes the reason to do it, with or without an audience, removing all aspects of the ego, stripping away the false image of our self and leaving us with the naked energy that the process generates.

Art is not a thing; it is a way. —Elbert Hubbard

In the realm of martial arts, the ego has become a powerful force, one that diminishes the purity of martial arts. It has always been the way. Even Myomoto Musashi, one of the martial arts legends of sixteenth-century feudal Japan, talked extensively about other schools that do not teach the Way in his book *The Book of Five Rings*. Too many martial arts styles focus on the body and become fixated upon the physical form, when in fact the truth lies in the spirit within. Yes, the body must be strong. (That is why we have the meditations of Chapter 2.) But the body is made stronger when the spirit is powerful; one's body is fed by the power that comes from a connection to something profound and universal.

This universality is the beauty of martial arts and of any art form. It applies to all things. This book is touching into something that is universal. It applies to all things. It is relevant to everything. Not to apply it to all things is to diminish what you are doing and your part in what you are doing. This connection to the "self" and to something greater can be achieved in everyday living. It does not have to be done in ancient Japan or ancient China (which is just as well). It does not have to be done through martial arts or some deep and meaningful teaching. It has to be done in the purity of the Way, the "do", or the Dao, to create a state of connection that brings us closer to the truth. The meditations bring us closer to the truth. We can meditate in business, at work, and at play. We can meditate in tennis, golf, and basketball. We can meditate in learning and in teaching. And we can meditate in music, art, and dance. The goal is to live a life of connection that in turn brings meaning to an existence that has no meaning.

Many ancient cultures understood that life has no meaning other than the meaning you yourself give it. The American Indians, the Australian Aborigines, the New Zealand Maoris, the Pacific Islanders of Fiji and Tahiti, the Inuits and Laplanders of the Arctic, the Incas, the Aztecs, the Druids, as well as the countless cultures of Asia and any of the World religions, all taught about a connection to the "Great Spirit" or something like it, that means we live to serve others as well as our own selves, knowing that to harm others harms us, and to harm us will harm others. That true meaning comes from walking a peaceful path, and sometimes that means we must fight to save the thing we believe in, to fight the struggles of life itself and discover our true potential, our true meaning, and our true purpose.

Confidence in our physical ability to defend ourselves gives us self-belief. It means we are less likely to walk through life in fear. The contracting energy of fear draws us into a shell in which our imagination plagues us with the perceived horrors life has to offer. In reality, more than ninety per cent of the things we worry about never actually happen, and we console ourselves by thinking that they might. Self-belief offers us the expanding feeling of trust and love. What do I have to fear? Very little, in truth. Things may be difficult and I may struggle, but that is not something to fear. That is something to overcome, and I will be the stronger for overcoming it. The limited scope of practical martial arts means that we are unlikely to use these skills face to face, so it is the confidence that these skills bring that sparks this expanding sense of confidence and power. If you have to use it practically, so be it, but even a warrior (a Samurai, a Viking, the SAS, or a Navy Seal) spends most of his life in a non-combative context. It is the man who in peace is haunted by his nightmares that makes himself a man of war. The true gift of martial arts is that a man is a man of peace always, a man who embodies the expansive energy of trust, love, peace, harmony, and tranquillity, a man who reflects the true essence of nature and the Universe, because he is the essence of nature and the Universe.

Man is made stronger by the struggles in his life. His spirit is tested, and the flames grow bigger as they feed on the trials of life. Any art creates obstacles and struggles. They place a mirror in front of us that shows us our strengths and weaknesses. We overcome, we persevere, we hone, and we practise until we master our self. The practicalities of the art are the means to strengthening the spirit so that we have the technical ability to express our self at that moment. Martial arts are no different in this regard. We practise forms so that we may enjoy the peace of "moving meditation" and become one with our self. The Japanese martial arts, to which I am most accustomed, are very specific about where things are placed, the path things take, and the positions of the body. Timing, tempo, and rhythm are intrinsic parts of the process. It is the same for all Japanese "-do". We learn this precision, which at first presents an obstacle to our learning, but in time we take these details into our being. No thought is required. We simply rest in the peace of the moment. This is the meditative state, and to perform in this state means we create beauty and tranquillity through our movement. We spar so that we may become one with our training partner so that we may in time become one with our enemy and realise that there is no separation, and that in turn leaves us to feel the experience of connection with all things. Read the words of the masters, Sun Tzu, Li Po, Chuang Tzu, Confucius, Lao Tzu, Jesus and the Gospels, Mohammed, Krishna, the chiefs and medicine men of the American Indians, Aborigine, Maori, and Inuit, Buddha, Moses, Shakespeare, Dickens, Aristotle, Marcus Aurelius, Thoreau, and many more wise men of human history, and you will see the commonality between them, the sentiment behind the words, the wisdom within the words, and the beauty between the words. The wisdom lies in the spaces, the rests, the silence, the gaps, and the nothingness, in "the sound of one hand clapping".

As a student of Zen and martial arts, I have struggled with this koan for many years, the idea of space and silence being the important part of things, the essence. Quantum physics supplies us with an explanation of this concept scientifically, while many cultures, including Buddhism, Hinduism, and Taoism, have spoken of this for millennia. Artur Schnabel said, "The notes I handle no better than many pianists. But the pauses between the notes, ah, that is where the art resides!" Truman Fisher said, "The pause is as important as the note." These quotes tell us that this wisdom is not restricted to martial arts. It is understood by many forms that wish to touch the very spirit of man. In the frenetic activity there is stillness, and in the stillness there is a space to move, to be, to become, and to grow.

Many years ago I saw a flamenco concert in London. With the passionate music of Andalusia, the young dancers jumped, leapt, and spun across the floor. With every move they stamped their physical authority onto the stage. It was very impressive. Later in the performance, an older lady came onto the stage alone to the delicate plucked notes of a Spanish guitar. She moved with none of the youthful vigour of the younger dancers, but she was mesmerising! Such grace, such passion, such power from within, and it held the audience spellbound. Sometimes she did not seem to move at all, yet it was perfect, in balance with the music and in harmony with the audience. It was as if her body had melted away, no longer on the stage, but a part of it. It was magic, the sort of thing that only comes with age, experience, and wisdom.

Just like the younger dancers of that flamenco troupe, in martial arts we assume we are solid—one solid object fighting another solid object. No wonder people complain about bumps and bruises in martial arts styles. It is a common thing. Even a trophy or prize in a competition or tournament is an expression of one's ego, a chance to demonstrate how tough one is.

I was taught a different way. If we can sense the fluid nature of our being, the lack of solidity, then we become something different, something lighter, faster, more effective, and more efficient. We feel before we are touched. We are aware at a different level, as if we are "seeing" waves coming towards us ahead of the physical body. These waves are connected to the physical body. Interact with the wave, and you affect the body. You interact with the wave by being sensitive to it. It requires you to "link" or to become aware of the other person in a nonphysical way, in the way of energy rather than in the way of the physical body. To be aware of this energy makes us sensitive to many things, not least the intent behind an attack, even what the attack will be and where it is focussed. But this works only with this link, for without it we are sensitive only to the next best thing, which is the visual physical separation that dominates our lives daily. It takes practice, for it requires a shift in our focus. We are used to interacting with the body, when in fact there is no need.

Practised in a safe environment where no harm can be done, we can hone the skill without fear, with confidence and a growing belief that what we are achieving is possible. For it requires belief. Any doubt leads to a sense of contracting energy, and then it cannot work. It is fluid energy interacting with fluid energy, and so it requires an expansive feeling or sensation. As we have discussed in the chapter on science, this fluid nature of being is reality. It is our focus on the solid nature of reality that makes the physical, bruise-inducing aspects of martial arts so real.

This different way requires constant awareness of the energy of people and things. My teacher talks about the fusing of one spirit with another, making the two as one. Then you move with your opponent without effort, even without touch. It becomes a thing of beauty, a dance rather than combat. In fact, ballroom dancing is not that much different to martial arts practised in this way. Combining energies generates flow but requires the surrender of the ego, the cessation of thought, and the lack of the need to win or the fear of loss. All is simply energy, and martial arts or any art form is the manifestation of that energy. Performed without ego, we can enjoy the feeling of fluid movement as it happens, without judgement, without self-consciousness, and without concern for anything at all. The motivation is the sensation. Without thought we are free to explore the endless possibilities that are truly available to us in the fluid nature of our nonphysical state. There is no sense of win or loss, only the sensation that comes in the moment itself. That is what the true artists seek to feel. A musician practises the same piece over and over again to hone his skill, but also because he loves the feeling of the flow of notes—the rhythm, tone, and timing, as well as the sound he makes. This is where the emotion lies, in the passion for his art.

In the Japanese and Chinese martial arts, both entwined with Zen and the Tao respectively, this concept of space and flow is an essential aspect of the deeper meanings behind the physical disciplines. We have to work with the physical body first, because we require the physical skills of martial arts as a foundation for the more advanced concepts. Just as a musician learns how to play his instrument or an artist or a sculptor learns to work with the tools of his trade, so in martial arts the student learns his basic techniques until they become a part of him. Once the techniques or skills enter his soul or his spirit, then he is free to use them to express his spirit, to express his very nature. As Henry Ward Beecher said, "Every artist dips his brush into his own soul and paints his own nature into his pictures." This is energy expressing itself through energy. In martial arts we practice forms that give the student the opportunity to hone his skill both physically and spiritually. It is this expression of self that shouts out in the spaces and in the silence of the movements, the rhythm, and the tempo.

All true art forms are the same, and life is the greatest work of art we will ever have the privilege of contributing to. By finding our voice, by making ourselves strong, and by connecting to the whole, we ensure that we can make a worthy contribution to life itself. This is the humble work of this book, and this is the purpose of martial arts.

Balance, Peace, and Harmony

Karate and all other martial arts are at the violent end of peace and harmony. It might seem at first strange that martial arts have been included as part of a book on meditation and energy. Why do people want to learn martial arts? Many people learn martial arts, and in some countries they are a fast growing activity. There are obvious pluses to learning any martial art: the increased fitness and the sense of strength and power that comes with learning, as well as a sense of raised self-esteem and self-worth. All of these things are positively desirable for anyone. We all need to be physically fit and feel that we have worth in the world; however, we don't all feel that we do. Life very often can rob us of our self-worth. Sometimes we can feel that we never ever had any self-worth or that we just do not have any right now. There can be many reasons for that. Sometimes material poverty, the location where we live, our ethnic or religious background, our gender, or any number of other differences can separate or exclude us from the people who surround us and make up our immediate community. So any pursuit that will address and remove these feelings, or at least help us to take back some control within the way we cope with these difficult issues, can only be a benefit.

There are some obvious drawbacks to any martial art. Particularly, they are all violent by nature and violence is their outcome. When we learn any martial art we are exploring the violent side of our own nature. It does no one any good, male or female, to be totally passive. We all have to live in the world as it stands and respond to all that comes in our direction. We all need to protect our own personal space and feel that we can stand up for ourselves and not be trodden on or downtrodden or, worse still, physically hurt. It does not matter how peaceful we are ourselves or how balanced we feel we are. There will always be those people who will wish to disturb our inner peace, not to mention our outer peace.

From that perspective martial arts are a wise choice, because as our skill increases in the practise of martial arts, we are able to defend our physical selves that little bit better. We all make the world in which we live. It is the sum total of the actions of all of us collectively that make the atmosphere and energy of the world. What we all think, do, and say makes our world. The more violence we display and project out to the world, the more violent a world we will live in. The thing that most humans wish for the most is peace, so if we all add violence to the world, how peaceful a world will we all live in? We make the world in which we live. Our actions do not just stay with each of us. Our actions have implications far beyond ourselves. All of our actions are ripples on a pond that we send out into the world, and eventually they come back to us. Maybe not directly but indirectly, they will return.

We are our own nurturers. We all nurture ourselves. Each and every input that we put in makes the person that we become. So if we put in nothing but violent inputs, it is likely that, unless we address that balance, we may become violent people and be desensitised to violence. We are modern man, and we live in civilised societies. Our societies are organised in such a way as to allow us reasonable free movement to go about our lives in a peaceful and ordered way. We do not need to club each other on the head to progress through life. For one thing, it is just plain impolite. It is not necessary and will only add to the lack of peace within society. What we put out to the world is generally what we get back from it. If we put out violence, then that is the world which we will inhabit. If we want peace, then we must put out peace, but we must realise that violence is indeed part of the human ability and is so for good reason. We have to keep that side of our nature in check, and the only people who can do that for us are ourselves. We must take charge of our emotions and actions and keep them in check. Meditation is at the other extreme to martial arts, and it will help to address the balance within the martial artist. It will bring the martial artist to a place of peace and thus help to balance the violent side of the martial artist's nature that is being cultivated by learning a martial art. It is well to remember that the outcome of learning a martial art is essentially to hurt people. Violence cannot be part of any modern civilised society that hopes to function with efficiency and human decency. Violence causes damage and pain, and that is not decent or efficient.

Life can be beautiful or it can be ugly. Whether is beautiful or ugly is up to all of us, the human beings who currently inhabit the earth. We make up human life on the earth currently. We are the only people who can make life beautiful or ugly. It all falls on our shoulders. If we put out disrespect and lack of love of our fellow man, then that is what will come back to us. If we act with love, respect, care, and kindness, then that is what will come back in our direction. There is nothing wrong with developing the violent side of our natures as it is a part of being human. What is wrong is to use that side of our nature to hurt others and to use that side of our nature to wreak havoc on our fellow man.

We are all of one family, the human family, and all people, no matter what you may or may not think or feel about them, have the right to life. They have the right to their life because they are here now and are alive. No one has the right to make less of that life for them. Equally, they do not have the right to act violently against you or disturb your peace. To own power and to never use it thoughtlessly, maliciously, or detrimentally is power indeed. That is a place of true balance. To cultivate that true point of personal balance, one must explore both sides of one's nature together in harmony.

If one side is explored and not the other, then imbalance can possibly ensue. To explore the passive side to the human nature and not the violent side is not as bad as the other way round, although it will possibly leave you a little vulnerable to life and to others. I am not in any way advocating that everyone needs to learn martial arts. What I am saying is that if you are learning them, then you will need in some way to keep your place of balance and peace. Also, if you do not acknowledge the violent potential of the human being, it could possibly lead to problems in your own life.

We can and should trust each other, but unfortunately not all people deserve our trust. Sometimes others are violent towards us, even if we have no such intention towards them. They may see us as vulnerable and weak in some way. Being able to deflect the possibility of violence is the desirable outcome to such a situation. To deflect violence we need to learn how to deal with violence.

I have an aunt who learnt self-defence when she was a young woman. She always enjoys a walk after her evening meal each day. One evening on her walk, a young man tried to attack her, and she threw him to the ground. He was so stunned that he could not move for shock. Even if we do not wish to learn how to do that, each of us needs to feel we can be assertive enough to keep our own place of peace and harmony. Violence in itself is not bad. However, using violence against another human being is bad, as it does not add to the sunshine and peace that we all crave so much. It does not add the beauty that we all deserve.

Violence Comes in Many Forms

Violence comes in many forms. Suffering is a part of life, and violence causes suffering. Violence is a complicated issue. I have heard many people say in recent times that they feel there is more violence in our society than in the past. I am not sure if there is or not, but at times it certainly does seem to me that there is more. I personally feel we are more accepting of violent acts and are becoming less shocked by them as they are reported more and more on a daily basis. I think that more violence is reported in the news. I am not sure if that means there *is* more violence in society or just that more seems to be reported. In both Britain and the United States there have been acts of violence in schools by pupils. We have all heard and read of these cases, I am sure. When I was at school some fifty years ago, such things were never known. This is a worrying and shocking new occurrence. Are we in the West becoming more violent and less feeling for the needs of others? Are we and our children losing our way and becoming more violent and accepting of violence? I hope not.

Violence is a natural condition of nature. Animals employ violence so that they may kill for food or protect themselves or their offspring from attack. It is a necessity as a means of survival. Even man must use violence to kill for food and to protect his personal safety. This is a part of the natural law. Where man differs from other creatures in nature is that he uses violence without benevolence. He uses it to gain power over others, to impart fear, to obtain dominance, or to abuse his position of trust so that he can have more than others. In short, it is for greed that man uses violence. It is for fear of demonstrating weakness that he employs ruthlessness. It is for fear of impotence that he is so savage. Savageness demonstrates a lack of trust among mankind, for if there were true trust between men, then there would be no need to be savage. To have true trust, there must be no fear. To have no fear, there must be a feeling of equality at some level.

The reason this is so important to our book about energy is because man uses the violence in his nature very often as a negative force, its need born from negativity and fear. How can we grow into the best versions of ourselves if we resort to violence brought about by fear? For fear is the ascendant feeling here—fear of being hurt, fear of being found out, fear of not being good enough or strong enough, fear of ourselves and of others.

We also know that people who have been violently abused in some way will often in time go on to become abusers and perpetrate violent acts on others. Criminal psychologists tell us that in part there is a desire on the part of the perpetrator to give back the pain that has been suffered by the perpetrator as a victim. Many people who are abused survive the ordeal by switching off their feelings. They become empty and numb. A chain of destruction develops that is passed one to the other. There are many kinds of violent abuse, mental, physical and sexual. All lead to a road of negativity and pain. The sufferer lives through the pain in many ways long after the initial attack takes place, and, as has been said, some go on to commit violent acts against others.

Lives are destroyed by these acts of violence. Our societies have to pick up the pieces of the destruction that is caused by such negative behaviour and interaction. A part of the purpose of life is to feel. We are spiritual beings as well as physical beings, and the spiritual side of us feels and connects to others. We empathise with each other. This is a necessary part of being human. It helps us to interact with each other and helps to protect our species.

Violence is promoted as an acceptable means for interaction by movies and video games that show it to an absurd degree. It is exciting, it sells (along with sex), but does it mean we are becoming desensitised to it? Is it okay to resort to violence, or does it show an increasing lack of emotional intelligence within society that we feel the need to resort to violence more and more of the time?

Daniel Goleman discusses this very social problem in *Emotional Intelligence*, a revolutionary book when it was first published in the 1990s, that is now well accepted as an issue for many people in society that resort to violence. They learn that violence is not the only way and that emotional articulation is an essential part of our development. Goleman discusses how violence often comes about through impotence, an inability to express how we feel or frustration at our situation in life, and through being shown that the best way to respond is to be violent. In short, violence as an interaction between human beings is taught behaviour that we learn. Do society and families have a responsibility to teach people kind and loving responses and interactions? I think so!

It seems to me that until people can be given the opportunity to feel empowered and to be supported to find their way in the world so that they feel they are doing something meaningful, the trend will continue to spiral downward towards greater violence. If a person feels equal and valued as an individual, he feels the power of his own being, and that is power enough.

To make a difference, people have to feel empowered. They must actually be in control of their lives rather than driven by invisible forces that take them to where they do not want to be. I may be naive, but I believe people fundamentally want to be good and to do something worthwhile with their lives. The only reason they do not do so is because they do not feel empowered to do so. The empowerment is value and resource. When people feel they have a true place in society and that they are valued and respected by others and in society and in humanity as a whole, then they are at peace. To be truly at peace with each other, these things need to be present.

This book is designed to empower its readers to seek the answers within and for you to help others seek the answers within themselves. The answers come not through the negativity of fear and violence, but through the positivity of self-knowledge and self-empowerment. It lies within us all.

Each and every Master, regardless of the era or place, heard the call and attained harmony with heaven and earth. There are many paths leading to the peak of Mount Fuji, but the goal is the same. There are many methods of reaching the top, and they all bring us to the heights. There is no need to battle with each other - we are all brothers and sisters who should walk the Path together, hand in hand.

—Morihei Ueshiba

How to Connect Consciously to a Person's Energy

There is a process in learning to connect to the energy of another person. Being consciously connected to another person energetically has many uses, and in martial arts it is a plus, and so I have included this exercise here. To connect to another person's soul, do the meditation that allows you to connect to other people. Just modify it a little by connecting to one specific person instead of all people. Have a look at meditation 2 of set 3 and modify it. It reads:

> Bring your attention to your own body. Now connect your spirit to others. Understand that you are one of many. Understand that you are connected at source.

Instead make that:

> Bring your attention to your own body. Now I wish to connect my spirit to . . . (Give the name of the person here.)

Just modify the words and ask for guidance to connect to the other person. You know how to do this in the depth of your soul. Just go into meditation and ask for guidance.

This meditation will give you a very close connection to the person, and you will feel the essence of that person. However, if you wish to just feel their energy, here are some exercises that will help you hone that skill. We have talked previously about how we can become one with our opponent so that we are part of them and they part of us. Everyone, including you, feels and connects to others on an energetic level whether we are consciously aware of it or not. At this stage of the book, you should understand how to bring energy down from the top of your head into your solar plexus. We have talked previously in the section of chapter 1 entitled "Energy Is a Big Subject" about how to bring down energy from the top of your head.

For those of you who have not read chapter 1 yet, here it is again more or less.

1. If you are still unsure about bringing the energy down, please imagine a ball of energy above your head.

2. Now with the power of your mind imagine that energy travelling down your body through your chakra points to the solar plexus. For any one unsure of where that is, it is the upper tummy area. Check the diagram that is in this book describing the chakras and their locations.

3. Imagine the energy at the size of a tennis ball and let it grow to the size of a beach ball.

4. Now that we have our beach ball of energy I would like you to send that energy out of your solar plexus into the room.

You probably did not feel anything, or if you are lucky you did. Most people don't the first time around. They do not connect into the energy or how it feels. This energy exercise is just helping you to experience the sensation of the energy consciously and manipulating it.

Now try this exercise with a friend sitting in front of you. Do exactly as I have described 'to you again. Bring the energy in from the top of your head, and bring it down the body through the chakra points to the solar plexus. Once at the solar plexus, grow the ball of energy to the size of a beach ball, and now send that energy strait out with force to your friend. Imagine really hurling that energy at them.

Don't worry. You are not going to hurt them in any way. It is only subtle energy. You will need to imagine hurling it at them to connect into their energy, as you are probably not used to manipulating the energy at will. Hurling the energy just helps you to feel something, as it will your friend. They too are probably not used to feeling this energy consciously, and so they will not feel it at first. Eventually you both will become sensitive to it and will feel the energy. It should not take many attempts for you both to feel the energy. Now swop over and have the other person do the exercise of throwing the energy at you. Once you feel the energy consciously, you will always do so. Do this exercise standing in front of each other, and have the person who is receiving the energy stand with their eyes closed. Watch what happens to them.

This is a very aggressive exercise to teach you to feel the other person's energy. It is one that I have found works. It was taught to me a long time ago, and I now teach it to my students. It helps them connect into the energy of another person consciously, maybe for the first time ever. We all feel each other's energy or aura all of the time. We just are not always aware that we are doing this.

Once you have mastered this exercise, practise sending your energy out to people gently and see what happens. I had a student whom I taught this exercise to some time ago. He was not convinced that we can feel each other's energy, and he decided to test my exercise. He told me that he walked a certain route each day and that at the same time and at the same point of the journey he would walk past a certain lady. He decided that he would throw his energy in her direction as he passed her, and as he did so she turned and smiled at him for the first time ever.

Maybe throwing your energy at unsuspecting people is not a good thing to do, but it will not hurt them if you have no intent of hurting them when you send it, and it will help you to learn to connect consciously to other people. If you send your energy out with harmful, intent they will feel that from you. Once you can feel the energy that you are sending and receiving, just send out the energy gently to the person, and with the power of your mind and thought just imagine bringing the energy back to yourself. Ask yourself, "What do I feel about this person?" not "What do I think about this person?" You should have an idea of how the person "feels" to you. To ask yourself, "what do I think" about the person will bring about a different result.

You can also connect to another person by expanding your aura. I think it is not easy to expand your aura when you do not know where your aura is situated within you. The exercise above will help you to connect to your energy and your aura easily with a little practise. In time you will not have to push energy out or think too hard about the mechanics of this. You will lock into the other person's aura or energy very easily at will.

The more you practice this, the better you will become at it, and, as my co-author has said, this is a great tool in the dojo to be able to use. To be one in the dojo is a good thing, but to be one with all people is even better. Eventually, if you practise this enough and try to feel the person and not just the energy, you will be able to do that. You will feel their feelings and their totality. Always remember that as you feel their energy, they too feel yours. We feel each other subconsciously whether we know we do or not.

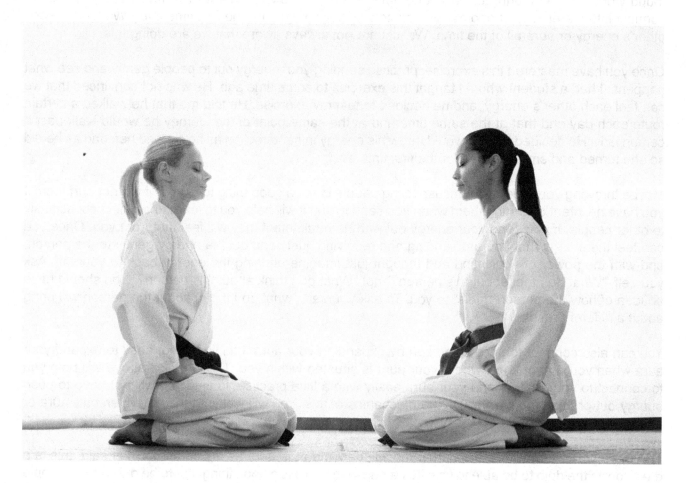

Go into your own peace, quiet and stillness and practise sending your energy out to other people.

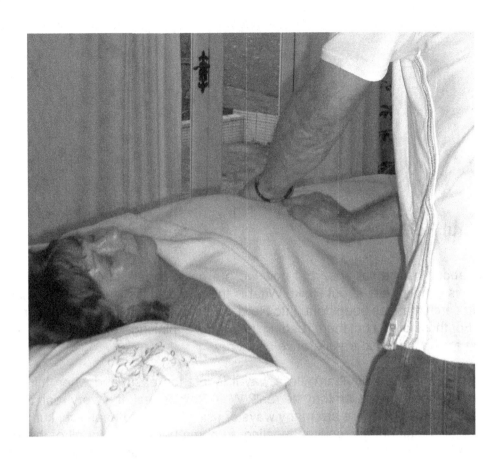

Reiki Precepts

Just for today do not worry.

Just for today do not get angry.

Honour your parents, teachers, and elders.

Earn your living honestly.

Be kind to every living thing.

Dr Mikao Usui

Reiki, Beautiful Reiki

We have talked about the martial arts, and now we are going to talk about the healing arts. Reiki, beautiful Reiki! This is how I feel about Reiki. What is there to dismiss about Reiki? There is a whole bucket load of research that has been done into Reiki. The results from that research are encouraging to say the least. For those of you out there reading this who are thinking, "What is Reiki"? I shall tell you. Reiki is a healing art that uses the transference of energy.

Reiki is so easy and it is so easily learnt. In a way it is just too easy, and when things come to us easily, we tend to question them. Can they be real? Well, Reiki is real. It is very real. Just as you and I are both real, so too is Reiki. There are many ways of using energy to heal—chi kung, acupressure, acupuncture, cranial sacral therapy, spiritual healing, to name but a few. Not all of these healing arts are exactly the same. Each in its way, however, is trying to bring back to the body its lost balance and harmony. When we lose our energetic balance, the body eventually responds with some form of physical ill health. We lose our energetic balance through being out of sorts emotionally. We can be overworked or overwrought with life's disappointments and pressures, and this in turn leads to us being out of sorts on the emotional level of our being. Emotional downturn within us can most often lead in turn to some sort of physical illness, unfortunately. I am talking about stress, the silent killer.

For centuries the peoples of the East have talked about energy—chi, ki, and prana. In the West we have for the most part dismissed their understandings and their take on life and health as superstitious rubbish. Things are changing in the West as the knowledge that the East has on this subject is being slowly taken on board by many. Now, how many of you out there reading this feel this way about the beliefs and understandings of the East? Hands up! I bet there are a good few of you. It is not easy to let go of what you are taught to be real and true.

When I was a young art student learning colour theory, I was told that we as artists do not have to reinvent the wheel, just tweak the design. So let's have some blue wheels or red ones or whatever as the fancy takes me as an artist or designer. I have come in on the story at a point where the wheel is in existence, and I do not need to invent it, just use it. This is also the case with healing and Reiki. It is there. It is out there, and all I need to do to use it is to tap into it. Now there lies the true problem and the six-million dollar question. How do I do that? How do I tap into that healing energy to enable me to bring well-being and repair to my body or the bodies of others? Well, within the Reiki community the "how" is a secret. It has been a secret that has been handed on from master to student since the beginning of Reiki healing therapy. So if you wish to learn Reiki healing, you must find a master to teach you. However, you can also tap into the Universal energy by doing the meditations within this book. The meditations in the health chapter of this book are a good place to start to tap into the Universal energy that will bring healing to you.

To find a Reiki master is easy. All you have to do is go the web site of the UK Reiki federation, or the equivalent of the Reiki federation in your country, and there you will be able to take your pick of who you wish to teach you. There are people out there, I am sure, who will perhaps trick you if you allow them to. Within Reiki, this is difficult. All Reiki people are traceable through their lineage. All Reiki people are traceable back to the founder of Reiki. In that there is a comfort, for you can ask to see any Reiki person's credentials. They will have certificates to say how they came about their Reiki knowledge and who passed that knowledge on to them. To do Reiki 1, there are no requirements other than the willingness to learn and to put aside scepticism for the duration of the learning process. There is a way that Reiki people use to bring to you the ability to be able to tap into the energy flow of the Universe and use that energy flow to bring healing on any and all levels of a person's being.

Now, for all of you people out there who think otherwise, this is not hocus pocus. I urge you to read *The Energy Healing Experiments* by Gary E Schwartz, PhD. Gary Schwartz is a professor of psychology, medicine, neurology, psychiatry, and surgery at the University of Arizona. This is an impressive resume by anyone's standards. *The Energy Healing Experiments* is a book to read cover to cover, for I am sure that what you will find in this book may well be a revelation to you.

I have an aunt who had her hand badly damaged in a car crash. It was set poorly, and now she has lost quite a bit of use of that hand. She also suffers from sciatica. When I phoned her one day, she seemed to me to be very poorly, and I enquired as to her welfare. She was in a good bit of pain. My aunt is a person who puts a good deal of faith into logic, science, and keeping her feet on the ground. She is not one for hocus pocus. I said to her that I would send her some absent healing. I am sure you can understand this did not impress her. However, she had been in so much pain for some weeks that if I suggested we cut off her offending hand and leg, she would have agreed. I sent her some healing that day and phoned her a few days later to see how she was, and she told me that all the pain had disappeared. It remained like this for about a week, and then the pain returned. So once again I sent healing, and the pain went away, only to return again in a couple of weeks. So we went on, my aunt and I. I sent healing and her pain levels improved, and then the healing dissipated and we were at square one again. My aunt looked for reasons for her improvement when I sent her the healing. She could not find any logical explanation at all. In time her sciatica went away, and, to be honest, I am not sure if she has suffered since. She has not mentioned it at all for a year or more.

Well, my aunt was curious and so I sent her a copy of the book by Gary Schwartz that I have mentioned to you. My aunt read it cover to cover and told me that she would like to be attuned to Reiki. Oh, I thought, now there's a thing! How was my logical and scientifically focused aunt going to take the explanation of attunement to Reiki? Hmm, I thought, and so I said yes, I would attune her, and we set a date. I did my attunement over the phone because it would have meant that one of us would have to travel across Britain just for the attunement. I sent her a manual. My aunt is a smart cookie, so I knew she would get the gist from the manual and she could phone me, and I would always be on hand to help. I thought that when we eventually met up at some point, we could go over all that she needed to know on the Reiki front if she needed to do so.

My aunt started on her self-healing twenty-one day period that is the requirement of Reiki, and she has never looked back since. She can take her own health into her own hands, and now any pain that she suffers can be managed with the use of Reiki. My aunt does not talk to me about pain any longer. My aunt used her Reiki ability on her daughter recently. Her daughter had an operation to remove a large growth from her stomach. My aunt's daughter is a research scientist, so getting her interested was not easy. I am not sure how my aunt did it, but she did. She set about giving her daughter regular Reiki treatments after the operation. I was minding my own business one evening getting ready to go to bed, when the phone rang quite late at night. It was my aunt's daughter phoning me to give me an account of what had happened to her with the treatment that my aunt had just given her. She was so excited and in disbelief. "Lynette", she exclaimed excitedly, "I felt it. I could feel heat, and my mother's hands were not touching me. I felt her hands with my hands, and they were cold, but I could feel heat"

This sort of result is very common with Reiki. The energy is transferred from practitioner to client, and that is how results occur. The energy can be hot or cold. The person might feel nothing at all, or they may just feel the energy travelling through their body. They can experience some mild pain in some circumstances, but that will be short-lived as the energy does its work. The energy works in a healing capacity, because that is what the *intent* of the practitioner is. It is also the intent of the client, as they have agreed to be given healing, and so that is what the energy does. The intent does not have to be conscious. It can just be subconscious also, and there will be no difference in healing outcome. There does not have to be any belief for Reiki to work. Reiki is part of us, just like air is part of us. We may not believe that air will keep us alive, but as long as we take it into our body, it will. I can believe whatever I want about air; it will still keep me alive.

It is the same with the Reiki energy. Belief is not essential. There does not have to be belief on any one part. We do not connect to spirit past (dead people) within Reiki practice, as that is spiritual healing and not Reiki. Of course, with spiritual healing we are indeed using the same energy to heal, but we are asking for spirit past to connect the healer to the healing energy and then to use the healer as a conduit to allow free energy flow to the patient. I have no problem with spirit past, as I am a medium, and so, of course, how could I? However, I have to stress this point as so many people are confused by it. We do not need spirit past to help us with Reiki. We just connect ourselves to the Reiki energy ray.

Reiki is just energy. If I talked to you about a colour ray, you would be happy about that, and for the most part you would understand what I was talking about. We all see colour and we all understand light. There is no difference with Reiki, in that it is energy just as light or air is energy. We do not see Reiki, but we can all feel it if we so choose to make the effort to do so. If we quiet our minds and bodies, we will feel it. We have to learn how to do this; that is all. We need to switch off the noise of the twenty-first century and sit with ourselves quietly. That is a big problem for most people these days, for where on God's green earth can we go where there is no noise? It is everywhere, drowning us out. We need to go into that space that resides within ourselves and then reach out to the wider Universe once the connection with ourselves is obtained.

The process is . . . I connect into my soul, and then I connect into universal energy, and now Reiki energy flows through me. With the intention added . . . . I now wish to use this connection for the highest possible good of the person. I wish to restore well-being and balance to this person.

Of course, the Reiki practitioner does not have to do this each time they conduct a healing session, as they are attuned to the Reiki ray and will connect whenever they wish to do so very easily. There is no hocus pocus, just connection to a force that we are part of and that is part of us. When we have a Reiki attunement, we are connected consciously and permanently. I cannot forget where I left the connection and fight to find it. I just know how to get to that place in an instant, and there we have lift off, so to speak. We can send out the beautiful Reiki energy as pleases us and the universe. We can sprinkle a little tinsel and glitter as we walk through life.

My aunt told me a story. She said that she was in the doctor's surgery for a check-up, and there was a little baby about six months or so old. He was crying and distressed. So too was the poor mother distressed, as she was worried about her baby. My aunt started playing with the child's feet to soothe him. In no time at all, the child had settled and was looking much better. The mother said that she could not understand the fact that her baby had settled. She wanted to know why her son was now at ease. He had been sickly for a couple of days, and she had not been able to appease him at all. He had remained unwell and had become worse, not better. My aunt played dumb and took her leave and left the surgery when it was her time to do so. The two ladies met again whilst shopping a few days later, and my aunt inquired about the well-being of the baby. "He is so much better," the mother said. "I just do not understand." My aunt told me that she had not intended to make the baby well, just to settle him. She laughed and said that she hoped that she had not made the baby so well that it was a wasted visit to the doctor's. My aunt found the whole situation amusing—that she had set about this turn of events with the baby. All Reiki practitioners have many such stories of healing great and small. Reiki is known to speed up the healing process and reduce pain. It has a very good track record in alleviating many illnesses. As I have said, it accelerates the healing process and allows our bodies to find that natural healing ability within. Our bodies know how to be well. They know what well is. When we cut ourselves, our skin heals. We do not have to think about it to make it happen; our bodies just do the work. It is that natural healing process that your body knows so well. Reiki encourages the body to its own natural well state. When your body is in a downward spiral health-wise, Reiki stops that in its tracks and sets in motion an upward turn.

Well, you can take what I have told you or dismiss what I have told you as rubbish. That is your choice. Make your own judgments by experiencing Reiki and not from the hearsay of others. Please do not take my word for the attributes of Reiki. Find out yourself. Try Reiki and then judge for yourselves. That is the best way to understand what is real and what is not. All Reiki practitioners will have a certificate and a lineage. They must be insured to work with the public, so that gives a little peace of mind. Reiki cannot harm you; it can only help you, and like all things, there are people practicing Reiki at varying standards. Just like any therapy, it is no different in Reiki. So find out who suits you best and who obtains the best results for you.

Enjoy Reiki. It is a tool that is your right as a human being to be able to tap into for your own health and well-being. It works on all levels of the person. It works on the emotional level of the person, the physical level of the person, the mental level of the person, and the spiritual level of the person. Use it also to bring harmony and balance within situations. Situations are made up of energy as well. People deal in situations, so we are working on multiple people when we work like this with Reiki. Reiki has many uses, and it is there for each of us—those who have the wisdom to pick it up and use it. Once you have learnt and understood Reiki, I am sure you will not look back.

The first three meditations of this book will strengthen your connection to the Reiki energy, so if you are learning Reiki or practicing Reiki, they are the meditations that you need to do to help you develop your connection and your skill. Reiki, beautiful Reiki! It is within me and it is outside of me. It transforms me and makes me well. It balances me and it helps to make me whole. It can and will do the same for you, if you allow it to do so.

Reiki Energy

How can you explain the feelings of the Universe? Can you explain the feelings of the Universe at all? Some years ago I decided to learn Reiki. Reiki is a traditional Japanese healing therapy. Reiki's healing method is energy-based. Reiki has swept through the West over about a seventy-year period. It came to the West a little before the Second World War.

When I decided to learn Reiki, I had no knowledge of what it was. I truly did not. I do not even remember what I supposed it was. I was as green about Reiki as one could be. I had just heard the word and knew that many spiritual people either could do it or aspired to learn it, and I suppose I thought it would be a good thing to do on the spiritual path that I was on.

I come from a background of a very logical and no-nonsense family, and this kind of thing was seen as a novelty to be tried at best. In fact, in my family when I was a child, if Reiki had been in our knowledge base at all (which it was not), it would have been seen as load of old rubbish. I am sure there are still many people out there in the world who will think that, despite a huge amount of evidence and research that is now saying things to the contrary.

It is easy to get sucked into other people's ideas, thoughts, and feelings. One can easily drift along on a tide of apathy and not question anything. It is good to think, and it is good to question. For it is in reason that we can determine what is real and what is useful to us and what is not. As a child of the fifties and sixties, and I grew up in the time when man first landed on the moon. I remember staying up all night with my mother and one of my sisters to watch the famous moon walk. I am not sure if we went to school the next day, but I suspect that my sister and I did not. I do remember writing about the experience of watching the moon walk in my diary the next day. It seemed so exciting to think that man had actually managed to do the one thing that was said to be impossible. Man had done it. He had conquered the ultimate impossibility. Surely now anything was possible for man to achieve. Logic and reason and a great deal of money and hard work would achieve everything and anything. Those were my thoughts at the tender age of thirteen. If we could go to the moon, we could do anything through logic and reason.

I understand the power of logic, and I have always used it in my life. At the times in my life when things seemed not to go correctly for me, I would always apply logic and reason to move myself forward in any given direction of my choosing or any direction that was necessary for me to go in. Logic has always served me well in my life. In my opinion, there is a great deal of good to be said for both hard work and logic. It is easy to dismiss anything as unreal if one wishes to do so, as all one would have to do is to say it does not exist. Once those words are said, we can turn off and turn away from that which we do not want to acknowledge. We can be ostriches if we so choose. We can close our ears and eyes to what is real, and we can bury our heads in the sand. If we bury our heads to that which we wish not to acknowledge, will that make it unreal? Well, of course not. If something is real and is in existence, then whether we choose to acknowledge it or not is neither here nor there. The thing is in existence, and to make it truly go away, we must physically destroy it.

My logical Western thinking has always served me well. There are many things in this world that we have no explanation for. Science looks at those areas that we cannot readily explain today in the hope that tomorrow we will add those explanations to our collective human knowledge base. We are curious creatures, we humans. That curiosity has served man both well and ill. Curiosity has brought man many useful answers that have in turn changed the course of history forever. We have tools, chemicals, machines, power, buildings, and design skills that have all been the results of curiosity and logical thinking. We equally have the means to destroy the earth many times over, and that too came about through man's logic and drive for knowledge and answers. Religious and esoteric thinking, knowledge, and understanding are most often dismissed in the West as superstitious rubbish.

There are three camps of thinking that are interesting to me. These are the religious, the spiritual, and the scientific. Obviously, not all people in any group think exactly the same or have exactly the same beliefs. There are always variations of thought, belief, and understanding. However, in most groups there will be an agreed body of knowledge and understanding that will be accepted in the main by the members of the group. I think that it is fair to say that. The religious camp of thinking is belief-based, the spiritual is experiential/belief-based, and the scientific are logical/experiential-based. Each approach has its merits. I do not believe any one of them is better than the others, just that each has a different approach to life's questions.

How does all of this tie into Reiki? We all think we know what is real, until something comes our way to challenge what we think we know to be real. We are given a way of viewing the world by society, and we are told what to think is correct and real. Not all people have the same experiences in life and reality. What I am saying about Reiki is that it challenges our perception of what is real and what is not. It has certainly challenged my perception. There are many things we think we know, but how much do we really know?

My Reiki journey started some years ago when one day I decided that I wanted to learn Reiki. I did not know what Reiki was. I only knew its name and that it was some sort of holistic healing practice. I thought it would be a good thing to learn. Although I did not know anything much about Reiki, I decided on a whim that I would learn it. In fact, I knew nothing apart from the name Reiki. I did no research about it at all, and on the very day that I decided that I would learn this holistic therapy, I went on the internet looking for someone in my area who would teach it to me. I found a lady in my area who was giving a talk on the subject the very next Saturday, so I emailed her and she invited me to come along, and so I did. She talked a bit about the history of Reiki and how it was energy healing, and this appealed to me as I did understand something about energy.

I have in recent years through my spiritual development come to learn many things about psychic energy. Psychic energy is the same as chi energy or ki energy. These names are just different names for the same form of energy. So that was it. I signed myself up for the course, and within the next few weeks I was being attuned. Now this was something that I did not get. I did not understand the attunement process. If I had learnt anything in the past, like most of you reading this, it was a matter of turning up for a lecture, listening to the information given, learning the information, and using the information. Attunements . . . umm, what were they? However, I went along with it all. On the day of attunement I was asked to sit with my eyes closed for probably twenty to thirty minutes. I sat there wondering what was going on around me and what was happening that would turn me into this healer like Jesus and Buddha. I must admit, I sat there thinking it was rubbish and asking myself why I was going along with it. I also remember thinking, "What if this is real and it does something terrible to me?" The teacher had explained that once I was attuned, that would be it. I would be changed forever and there was no going back. The process could not be reversed. As I sat being attuned, I thought about this, and there was a part of me that was totally unsure about signing up for something so permanent, even though I did not truly believe it was going to work.

To say that there was a bit of confusion in me is putting it mildly. It was a bit like being split in two directions. On the one hand there was my Western logic telling me this was a load of old rubbish. On the other hand there was the side of me that was energetically aware that was saying, "Go for it!" Well, the first attunement was done and dusted, and I had survived it. The teacher asked for any experiences. I did not really have any except for a bit of a sore head. The top of my head felt mildly sore. The teacher had not touched my head, and so that was a little curious. I brushed that entire experience aside and listened to my classmates relaying their experiences of coloured lights and feeling energy and seeing this or that.

We practised healing on each other during the day. I lay on the couch, and the classmate who was assigned to me gave me Reiki healing. For those of you who do not know what that is exactly (as I did not in those days), as I said at the beginning of this chapter, it is a Japanese healing therapy that is energy-based. This method of healing is thought to go back thousands of years to the time of Buddha and Christ. Who knows if it does or not? It may well do. However, that is not the point. The point is that it uses energy. It uses an energy that is around all of us and is part of all of us. This energy is the energy of the universe. It is called universal life force energy. Or in other words ki, chi, or psychic energy. It is an electromagnetic energy that is part of us all.

I have to admit I did feel something in that healing. I had been convinced that I would not. I did indeed feel energy from the student healer to me. When it was my turn to heal, I felt energy in both of my hands and being transferred to the student patient. I did question what I felt, but I knew that I did in reality feel something. It took me much more time than that initial first weekend to finally put aside my doubts about Reiki. I did my Reiki 2, the professional level, and have since that time gone on to become a Reiki master. I have had some impressive results with my healing, and I am both proud and pleased to have been able to give some help to others at a time of need. Reiki 2 brought a whole new set of doubts and fears. At this level of Reiki the student is introduced to three of the four Reiki symbols. This was another test for my Western logic, and this level saw me once again doubting the teaching and knowledge of Reiki. How can symbols evoke healing in anyone? This question left me huffing and puffing and a bit cold. Surely it is not possible to send healing to another person? How can we do that? How can a symbol be anything other than marks on paper? My logic told me that it was not real and it was not possible.

I was taught to pick up the energy from the paper via the symbol drawn and post it to one of my classmates. My classmate sat opposite me. They said they felt the energy, and once again I thought, "What's going on here? This cannot be real." When it was done to me, I could feel the energies and the quality of those energies. My first two Reiki levels were a challenge and an eye-opener for me. I have since that time been so grateful to whatever gave me the thought to learn Reiki.

Now, as I have said at the beginning of this discussion, it is so easy to dismiss anything that does not fall into our own personal experience and understanding as rubbish. I have been guilty of that myself. Of course we must not lose our powers of reason and logic; they must be preserved at all costs. However, to dismiss out of hand ideas and thoughts as rubbish without proof that they are rubbish is maybe just a little short-sighted, to say the least.

My belief now is that Reiki is real, and my experiences with Reiki have given me that understanding. To find my place of acceptance of the truth and reality of Reiki in my personal understanding took two years of my life or thereabouts. I did not come to Reiki through a sense of initial belief or disbelief or knowledge, just a whim. Maybe that was the right way for me, because I suspect that if I had done some research, I would have not gone in Reiki's direction, and my life would have been the less for that.

I am grateful to the founder of Reiki, Dr Usui, who bothered to search for the knowledge of Reiki and also to the others who send it to the West. I hope that Reiki travels to all four corners of the earth and helps as many people as Reiki needs to help. I would like to see a day when it is the accepted norm for this healing method and others like it to be used in our hospitals, along with conventional Western medicine. That day has begun, and now there are hospitals even in Britain that are using Reiki to help their patients.

There has been a great deal of interest in Reiki in recent years, and research on Reiki is happening in various countries. One has merely to go on the web to find those countries and places where research is taking place currently. Dr Gary Schwartz has published a book containing the results of his research into Reiki, as I have previously said.

Change is always slow, and the change in the tide that has for so long made up Western thinking is especially slow. As much as I am a medium and a Reiki practitioner, I am also an artist and a designer, since that too is part of my training and knowledge base. In art and design one needs to use the power of reason and logical thought to create beauty through intuition. That observational and logical and expressive approach to life was encouraged for ten years of my life. That is as much part of me as any esoteric training and knowledge that I have. All of those ideas and approaches go to make me myself. I find that one sits alongside the other very nicely, thank you. As I have explained, it did not always do so, and I had to go on a personal journey with Reiki, as well as the other areas of spiritual and energy work that I have also learnt and developed.

The bottom line is this: we are all energy, and this is something science agrees upon. We are part of the universe; this too science agrees upon. The universe is energy, and science also agrees with that notion. We are conscious energy, and we also have an interaction with all life and the wider Universe. We are energy interacting with energy. The Universe is us and we are it. We are a product of it. I can move air by bringing air into my body and expelling it. So why would I not be able to direct energy consciously and purposefully towards another person? Why is that so impossible? Just because a thing is outside our ability to prove it or is outside our personal knowledge base does not mean it is not real. It just means that the majority of people so far in the mainstream of thinking cannot prove it to their personal satisfaction as fact.

I have witnessed through my life many changes in thinking and belief. When I was a child, it was accepted by the majority in Britain that the thing to do was to be a good Christian. To be a good Christian one had to go to church on Sunday and say one's prayers each and every night. Today, our Christian churches are emptying and closing one by one. Most of society is not going to church. There has been an increasing shift towards Eastern philosophy or no philosophy at all. One has just to look at the goods in any department store. There are so many plastic Buddhas for sale or Buddha pictures. I have no opinion about this at all. I am merely observing the tide of change and commenting on that observation.

We are in some measure becoming open to change and new possibilities. This increases our knowledge base, and in turn we move forward with those new understandings. For the better or the worse, who knows? That is perhaps dependent on ourselves and how we wish to use new knowledge. I started by asking, "How can you explain the feelings of the Universe?" Well, by connecting to the Universe and feeling what it is feeling, of course.

The Wealth of Knowledge on Reiki and Health Benefits

It is not my intention to add to the wealth of knowledge that is available on the subject of Reiki itself. At the end of this book you will find a list of titles that you can read that will help you understand what Reiki is in more depth. It is just my intention to share with you the reality of Reiki and my personal experience. There has been much research into Reiki in recent years, and this research, I think, is causing some people to wake up and wonder. The meditations within this book can only enhance your Reiki practice if indeed you do already practice Reiki. That is the intention of this book—to give you enhancement on your Reiki journey and to give you, the practitioner and the non-practitioner, the understanding that Reiki is energy that is freely available from the universe. It is part of the fabric of your being, and the practice of Reiki therapy harnesses and uses this energy for healing purposes. We all have an innate ability within us to heal ourselves and others. Most of us are just unaware that within ourselves exists the ability to heal. To go on a journey and look for something, we first have to at least find a place within our being that will allow us to accept the possibility of the existence of that thing. If we do not believe that it exists or at least believe in the possibility of its existence, we will not look for it. So if we are too sceptical about new possibilities, we will stand still and never move forward. We must at least be open for a short while to have a look at the possibility of something.

The meditations in the book will enhance your existence in this life and give you a deeper connection on all levels of your being. This connection has many uses, and your practice of Reiki will benefit from the deeper connection that will reside in you as you do the meditations and develop that deeper connection to the universal energy.

Some of the Benefits of Reiki
- It accelerates the body's self-healing abilities.
- It will support the immune system.
- It can help M.E. and energy levels.
- It can help headaches.
- It creates deep relaxation.
- It aids the body to release stress and tension.
- It aids better sleep,
- It can help to reduce blood pressure

- It can help with acute injuries.
- It helps relieve pain.
- It helps to bring the body into balance and harmony.
- It helps to assist the body in cleaning itself from toxins.
- It aids the breaking of addictions.
- It can help eczema.
- It reduces some of the side effects of drugs.
- It helps the body to recover from drug therapy after surgery and chemotherapy,
- It can help Asthma.
- It helps Cancer.
- Reiki enhances and supports other healing practices and can be used alongside other holistic practices and conventional medicine also.
- Reiki helps the person take control over their own physical, mental and emotional health.

There are so many benefits to Reiki. The above are just a few of them. Reiki never harms, and it always helps and supports the person, their health, or the situation. There are no side effects to using Reiki. It seems such a shame with all of this in mind and with the recent studies and understandings about Reiki that more people do not know of it and use its benefits. Just the fact that it is superb at relieving pain and speeding up healing is alone a good reason to enjoy the benefits of Reiki. Reiki is just a beautiful healing energy that is part of the person's being, and so there seems no reason not to use it to good effect. There is an awakening to Reiki, but it is slow. More and more people are finding and using the benefits of Reiki, but not enough in my humble opinion.

> "Believe nothing because a wise man said it.
> Believe nothing because it is generally held.
> Believe nothing because it is written.
> Believe nothing because it is said to be divine
> Believe nothing because someone else believes it.
> But believe only what you yourself know to be true."
>
> *The Buddha*

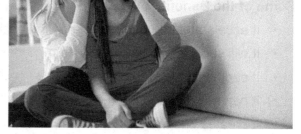

Conclusion

Now it's time to say goodbye, and we hope you have enjoyed the book.

A Final Note from Lynette.

To understand your life and what you are, know that the ancient peoples of earth understood a fundamental truth of life. They understood that you must indeed look to and observe life itself to find the answers to living.

They understood that there were elements to life that were greater than themselves. They regarded, revered, and worshiped the greater elements of life. We, the modern people of earth, have no such reverence on any level of our being for life on earth or within the universe. We have become sickly with our own personal power, and life is no longer a wonder to us. To understand your life you must have awe and wonder, for you are indeed part of a greater whole and you are indeed part of the magic. The magic of life exists on all levels of life. It starts with you but does not end with you. You are the Universe because you are made of the universal ingredient that is all important to life. You are made of the stuff of God and the stars. You are made of energy.

You are energy on all levels of your being—as is God, and as are all things. To revere God is to revere the wonders of all that exists within and without this life and possibly all life. Science is not really at odds with God; it is merely trying to explain what God is. Energy, both on a minute level and on a gigantic level, is energy. It interacts with energy. It is that interaction that impacts other forms of energy. It is said that we are made in the image of God. What if that image is energy itself? Would that make God any the less or us any the more?

We are energy with consciousness, and we have the capacity to consciously interact and impact other forms of energy. We have a great responsibility placed upon our shoulders as that consciously interacting energy form. We can create energy waves with the power of our minds followed by physical action. We have the capacity and the power to make choices that will change our lives and the lives of others and in turn our world and maybe other worlds and out into the wider universe, for we do not know how far our influence upon energy reaches. Does our influence merely extend to the earth, or does our influence, without our personal knowledge, impact upon other worlds far beyond ours? We know for sure that our own impact on our own world is great, and we are globally, nationally, and personally getting it far, far wrong.

We have the capacity to put things right, but we choose not to do so, for it is materially profitable for the majority of us in the short term not to do so. We sell, interact, consume, barter, exchange, and force upon others that which damages us in the long term for short term benefit. We are killing our own world and ourselves—spiritually, morally, and physically in the pursuit of a dream that is taking us all on a road to nowhere. We are the nowhere peoples of earth.

However, perhaps it is also true that there is now a slow awakening in the world today. Maybe this humble book is part of that awakening. The awakening is opening the understanding of all of us that much is in our own power. To exercise power we must first understand that there is power, that we are part of that great power that exists both within ourselves and without ourselves, and that we can connect to it consciously at will.

This new understanding is in reality old knowledge that illustrates that this power is multi-dimensional and can be harnessed and used for many things. We can use this power to develop our own inner spirit, our understanding, our physical bodies, our relationships, our personal lives, those of others, and our world. The first step on this road of change is to connect to this great power, and you have now taken the first step. The more you connect to this power, the deeper your connection will become. Repeatedly doing the first three meditations in this book will serve you well on your journey. Repeatedly doing all of the meditations in this book will serve you even better. We suggest that you meditate on all that we have shared with you in this book, for you are now well on your way to the pot of gold that is at the end of this journey. Enjoy!

A Final Note from David.

So, we have been on a journey. From wherever you were at the beginning of the book, you have been introduced to and have experimented with tools that have opened your perception to something greater.

The logical, analytical, left side of the brain cannot touch what the intuitive, creative, right side of the brain is in touch with all of the time. As creatures capable of consciously working with energy, we have the ability to quieten the left side so that we can explore this powerful and wonderful universal force with the right side. It opens us up to self-healing, self-understanding, self-exploration, and self-fulfilment, and it brings us to access the universal wisdom available to all. We may then be able to understand that which is beyond our left-brained intellect.

Moreover, this is an endless, constantly unfolding journey. When we begin, we touch the tip of the iceberg. As we grow, as our power grows, as our abilities allow us to penetrate more deeply into the void, the wisdom becomes greater, our power stronger, our self-belief more assured, and our inner voice louder.

We become more and more a force within our own lives, an advocate for our own potential, a positive force in our own lives and the life of others. As your perception grows, you may find the meditations become more profound. You will tweak them to fit your own feeling and your personal journey. Nothing is set in stone; all is feeling; all is about intuition.

We hope you have enjoyed what you have discovered and will continue to enjoy discovering new and exciting things about yourself, about others, and about life itself. After more than twenty years of self-discovery, we are amazed at what we find within us. Your journey will be different, but no less amazing.

To nourish the flame within . . .to keep the flame burning . . . we suggest you meditate on it.

A human being is a part of a whole, called by us 'Universe', a part limited in time and space. He experiences himself, his thoughts and feelings as something separated from the rest . . . a kind of optical delusion of his consciousness. This delusion is a kind of prison for us, restricting us to our personal desires and to affection for a few persons nearest to us. Our task must be to free ourselves from this prison by widening our circle of compassion to embrace all living creatures and the whole of nature in its beauty. Nobody is able to achieve this completely but the striving for such achievement is in itself a part of the liberation and foundation for inner security."

—Albert Einstein

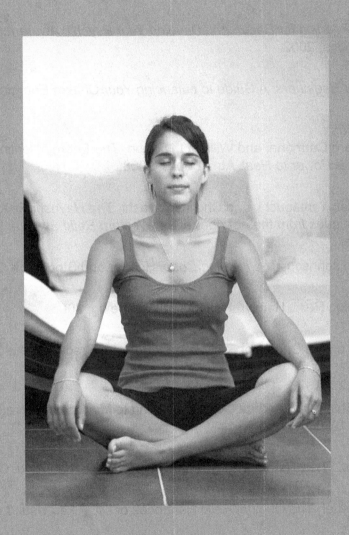

Condolence letter to Norman Salit upon the death of his daughter, March 4, 1950

Further Reading

Energy

Anne Jirsch and Paul McKenna. *Instant Intuition: A Psychic's Guide to Finding Answers to Life's Important Questions.* Paitkus, 2008.

Cyndi Dale. *The Subtle Body: An Encyclopaedia of Your Energetic Anatomy.* Sounds True, 2009.

Healing

Cassandra Eason. *Aura Reading.* Piatkus, 2000.

Richard Webster. *Aura Reading for Beginners: Develop Your Psychic Awareness for Health & Success.* Llewellyn Publications, 2002.

David Pond. *Chakras for Beginners: A Guide to balancing Your Chakra Energies.* Llewellyn Publications, 1999.

Gary E. Schwartz, Richard Carmona, and William L. Simon. *The Energy Healing Experiments: Science Reveals Our Natural Power to Heal.* Atria Books, 2008.

Frank Arjava Petter, Tadao Yamaguchi, and Chujiro Hayashi. *The Hayashi Reiki Manual: Traditional Japanese Healing Techniques from the Founder of the Western Reiki System.* Lotus Press, 2003.

Alexander Loyd and Ben Johnson. *The Healing Code.* Hodder and Stoughton, 2010.

Eleanor McKenzie. Healing Reiki. Hamlyn Health and Well-Being, 2005.

Tadao Yamaguchi. Light on the Origins of Reiki: A Handbook for Practicing the Original Reiki of Usui and Hayashi. Lotus Press, 2007.

Michael Bentine, Betty Shine, and Anthea Courtenay. Mind to Mind: The Secrets of Your Mind Energy Revealed. Corgi Books, 1990.

Betty Shine. Mind Waves: The Ultimate Energy that Could Change the World. Corgi Books, 1994.

Mikao Usui and Frank Petter. The Original Reiki Handbook of Dr. Mikao Usui. Lotus Press, 2000.

Deepack Chopra. Quantum Healing Exploring the Frontiers of Mind /Body Medicine. Bantam New Age Books, 1989.

Bronwen and Frans Stiene. The Reiki Sourcebook. O Books, 2003.

J.R. Worsley. Talking about Acupuncture in New York. Worsely, Inc, 2003.

Life

Martin E.P. Seligman. Authentic Happiness: Using the New Positive Psychology to Realise Your Potential for Lasting Fulfilment. Nicholas Brealey Publishing, 2003.

Erich Fromm. The Art of Loving: Classics of Personal Development. Thorsons, 2010.

Eckhart Tolle. The Power of Now: A Guide to Spiritual Enlightenment. Hodder & Stoughton, 2001.

Daniel Goleman. Emotional Intelligence: Why it Can Matter More Than IQ. Bloomsbury, 1996.

Fritjof Capra. The Tao of Physics. Shambhala, 1977.

Stephen R. Covey. The 7 Habits of Highly Effective People. Simon & Schuster, 2004.

Jonathan Haidt. The Happiness Hypothesis: Putting Ancient Wisdom to the Test of Modern Science. Arrow Books, 2007.

Tim Allen. I'm Not Really Here. Hyperion, 1996.

Viktor E. Frankl. Man's Search For Meaning: The classic tribute to hope from the Holocaust. Rider, 2004.

Annette Simmons. Quantum Skills for Coaches. Word4Word, 2009.

Meditation

Barry Long. Meditation: A Foundation Course - A Book of Ten Lessons. Barry Long Books, 1996

Contact

Lynette Avis

The Living Energy Studio

www.thelivingenergy.co.uk

email: lynette@thelivingenergy.co.uk

David Brown

www.potentialitycoaching.co.uk

Janette Marshall

www.janettemarshall.com

email: info@janettemarshall.com

About the Authors

Lynette Avis

Lynette is a graduate of the Central St Martin's School of Art. She trained at many top British art schools. Lynette is trained in interiors, fashion textiles, soft furnishing, and painting and drawing. She has always had creative ability and is a very skilled dressmaker and needle woman also. Lynette loves colour and the ways in which we can use colour to impact our lives. She is also interested in colour theory and is skilled in the use of colour within painting and within interior decorating. Lynette trained as a specialist decorator, which developed further her use of paints and the effects that can be created with colour and texture. She has renovated many properties, which has allowed her to use her many skills. Lynette became ill with M.E. and suffered long term ill-health; it was this that took her on a new and different path. She embarked on a spiritual journey to find answers for her poor health. Lynette was introduced to the world of mediumship and found she had ability within that. She has been a developing medium for many years and now is a teacher of spiritual development, psychic development, mediumship, and Reiki at her Living Energy Studio. Her exploration into subtle energy has further led her to qi kung in which she is a student. Lynette has been learning karate for many years, and it was in karate that she met her co-author David Brown.

David Brown

With twenty-two years of martial arts and self-development experience, David is also expanding into the arena of life coaching and mentoring. A thriving martial arts and self-development business allows him to explore many areas relating to personal growth, including Zen and other forms of self-knowledge and understanding, including practising meditation and studying ancient teachings of traditional cultures. David has two science degrees and has a number of published papers to his name. He continues researching his interests in science, including neurobiology and quantum physics, and using that to develop his approach to martial arts and life coaching.

About the Book

How can a book bring martial arts, meditation, quantum physics, Reiki healing, health, well-being, and one's place in the world together and explain them in a way that highlights their connection and uniqueness as part of a universal whole? Here we describe the essence of what binds the universe together and connects these seemingly disparate things—energy. We discuss how energy is the root of all these things and how we can harness its great power and potential to create lives for ourselves that are empowering, exhilarating, loving, and filled with a sense of awe and a desire to explore and discover … the way life is meant to be!

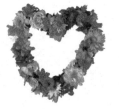